The Magic of Facial Exercise

Cynthia Rowland

The Magic of Facial Exercise

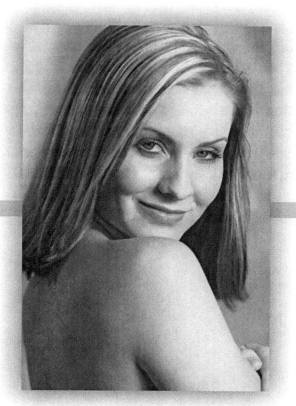

ALL ABOUT NATURAL BEAUTY

Book cover and interior design by Bookcovers.com

Published by:
Rejenuve, Inc.
P.O. Box 3902
Long Beach, CA 90803
www.cynthiarowland.com

ISBN 978-0-578-04669-3
Printed in the United States of America

DISCLAMER
This health information is solely for educational purposes and is not intended to replace your physician nor is it a prescription of medical advice. Application of this information is at the reader's own risk; this information is intended to be discussed with the reader's physician to determine the appropriateness and applicability. If you have a pre-existing medical condition or are currently under a physician's care or are taking medication, do not change or discontinue the recommendations of your physician without his/her knowledge. Take this book to the doctor with you.

Acknowledgements....

So many people have touched my life, believing in my vision to bring this information to all who want to capture the fountain of youth. Here are a few of my top picks...

I am indebted to Howard Harmon who has provided such incredible support with many wonderful years of friendship, love and companionship.

Marlene Hartsman, the "sassiest" woman I know who suggested years ago that I write articles and a book.

Sharon Shelton, a most interesting woman who loves me unconditionally and always has a dazzling smile to share with the world. She keeps my spirits high!

Gloria McMillan, my right hand gal, who stuck with me through the edits and rewrites, without complaining while interfacing with Karina Castrejon and Jennifer Nguyen to keep our office running smoothly.

Lynn Nielson/Larry Brandon, a dear couple who has given me heartfelt encouragement to succeed throughout the years.

Nina Nichols, a long-time friend whose great beauty is astounding and her love for life infectious; she is a dear, wonderful woman!

Connie Benesch for encouraging me to "let it out"!

Jackie Silver, my Ageless Sister, whose vision and inner strength provides me with confidence (I deeply love and accept myself) so that I understand that I am stronger than my fears.

Steven Tassopoulos, many thanks to you, my long-time fabulous friend for holding my hand and keeping me sane throughout the years with lots of love and laughter.

Table of Contents

Baby Boomers

Beauty

Botox

Career

Cheeks

Chin

Eyes

Facelift

Jowls

Lips

Look Younger

Men

Natural

Plastic Surgery

Sagging Face

Seasonal

Skin

Introduction

Hello, my name is Cynthia Rowland. You may recognize my name and my face from my many television appearances. I am a facial fitness expert and the creator of Facial Magic, the exercise program that has transformed many faces across the globe.

I learned of this exercise program when my friend Taylor told me that she had discovered a small clinic in Denver, Colorado that specialized in natural facelifts, and that I needed to get there right away. How did this happen?

My eye lid was sitting on my eyelash.

It did not occur overnight; in fact, the downward slide was sly and insidious. At first I did not recognize what was happening. My eye makeup was the primary clue. Mid-morning my mascara was showing up under my eyebrow like a dark shadow; how did it get there?

Several ideas came to me; when I looked into the mirror with my face relaxed. I could see a droopy eyelid. When I applied my mascara my eye brows elevated and my mouth opened. Hmmmm. You may do that too – it seems impossible to apply mascara with a closed mouth.

Bottom line – I had a droopy eyelid, my first sign of aging and there was only one remedy that I knew of. I knew it was not for me.

Taylor convinced me that I should immediately come to Denver. I hoped she was onto something but I had my reservations because it seemed unlikely that if something so wonderful was available, why had I not read about it in the news?

Thank goodness I flew to Denver to see with my own eyes the results of an exercise program that really, really works. Taylor personally took me to the clinic to meet the staff and I was intrigued from the beginning. The people there were dressed in professional attire, passionate about their work, promoting better health with something new: Facial fitness.

The staff introduced me to women, their patients, who were willing to show me their beginning photos. It was evident to me that their faces were indeed different! I could easily see lifted cheeks and eyes and their faces looked toned. I was terribly excited and wanted to learn the exercises myself! Right then!

Marcelle, a wonderful woman from France who guided her clients with enthusiasm and love, told me that my eyelid was not a problem – the look was caused when our eye brows that drop with age and then she zinged me by saying that the exercises would even help the little wattle I was developing. Wattle? I didn't even realize that the area under my chin was sagging, too.

My week-long trip to Denver turned into a 15 month odyssey. I worked daily at the clinic for over a year to learn how isometric exercise and resistance training can indeed re-shape and contour faces. It was an amazing time for me. I knew that these exercises deserved to be available for everyone, especially as my face began to look younger and younger.

Did I mention I was only forty?

Now, fast forward ten years: A few years ago the exercise program became available on video and the process, now a system—**Facial Magic**.

I love sharing the knowledge of facial fitness and hope you enjoy this book. The Facial Magic video system provides detailed information and writing this book allows me to enhance the information in a more comprehensive manner.

The Facial Magic regimen is fantastic for restoring muscle tone to the face and neck. You know the look: no matter how much rest you have had, you still "look" tired. Maybe strange things have begun happening to your face; maybe it is moving in a Southerly direction and there are hollows and indentations developing practically overnight.

Sometimes we look into the mirror and wonder *what happened* to that face we used to know? *How* and when did the drooping and sagging develop and what can we do to stop it?

It seems to me that the day we discover facial aging is the day we begin to notice all of our flaws and even claim more bad hair days. We have done everything we can do topically: cleaning, moisturizing, exfoliating and yet we see Mother Nature taking her toll.

Muscles in the face can elongate up to 50% by the time we reach our mid-fifties, so is it any wonder that we wear pools on our jaw line and have droopy upper eyes that make us look tired yet we feel so young inside? Our face, the first thing people see, can blatantly shout that we are wearing the ravages of stress, gravity and atrophy. We can cleverly disguise our body with long jackets, black slimming pants, etc., but our faces are different. Unfortunately, we cannot mask facial droopiness with a new hairdo, makeup or special creams.

Age usually is not bothersome; it's <u>aging</u> that can be almost overwhelming. Is it possible to do something short of surgery to correct those unwanted lines and the underlying problem of muscle atrophy?

We're sophisticated. We know that "miracle creams" can certainly smooth out lines temporarily but there is only one way to non-surgically correct the aging process that results in sagging muscles that create lines and wrinkles. That is exercise. FACIAL EXERCISE!

Facial Magic is a facial exercise program designed to enhance your appearance and give you greater confidence. How? When you take charge of your face, you give yourself the opportunity to restore the toned, lifted look you had when you were younger! When you feel positive about your appearance, I know you will have greater confidence in yourself.

There are added benefits to this program such as better posture and improved skin tone. With Facial Magic you can exercise those hidden muscles and drop years from your face easily, without going to a gym or buying special workout clothing.

I can't promise that you will look sixteen again; however, if you want to drop ten to fifteen years from your face in the next three months and change the look of your face, you first have to increase the strength in the muscles underneath the skin. After a few short weeks of exercise, your face will take on a fresh, improved look. Think about it…if you didn't move your arm for years, it would hang limply. The same applies to the muscles of your face.

You are never too old or too young to participate in this program. Just as you appreciate the good feelings in your leg and arm muscles when you do leg lifts, weight train, run or bicycle, the muscles in your face respond the very same way. Your face will feel revitalized and refreshed from the very first day you begin this program!

Facial muscles are much smaller than most muscle groups and experience tells me they rehabilitate easily. Every woman and man that I have personally supervised received very pleasing results using Facial Magic. Most muscles in the face are attached to skin and this program will teach you how to successfully work with these muscles so that you will achieve a more youthful face. Your skin will become vibrant and healthy looking, too.

Facial Magic introduces two exercises at a time so muscles strengthen slowly yet deliberately. In a few weeks, you will be working all areas of your face and neck and experiencing a toned, contoured and a lifted appearance.

Resistance training and isometric contractions will produce smoother skin and a healthier glow from increased oxygen and blood supply to the facial area reducing puffiness due to edema (excess water accumulation) as well as hollowness and other symptoms of muscle atrophy.

This book is a compilation of articles that I have written to provide you with very valuable information so that you can take control of your face. My passion is Facial Magic because it works!

Now let's create a love affair with your appearance....

Special Report
The Evidence Does Not Lie

It is easy to understand the confusion that occurs when a journalist or medical professional researches "facial exercise". There are literally hundreds of thousands of websites dispensing misinformation that scrunches, twitches, puckers and facial contortions are considered facial exercise. Blur that with non-surgical facelifts disguised as facial massage, devices in the mouth, electro-stimulators, even topical creams and invasive injections, it's no wonder there is mass confusion with no clarity when researching "facial exercise".

The 21st Century dawned with staggering statistics of desperate people using surgery and injections to enhance their appearance. The media has accommodated the drug companies and doctors by providing magazines, television shows and other outlets with an ongoing smorgasbord of invasive and not-so-invasive procedures and prescriptions paraded almost daily in sensationalized headlines and advertising. This deliberate brainwashing has lulled the masses into believing that invasive, risky procedures are the only way to reverse the signs of aging in the face.

> **...THE MEDIA HAS MISSED THE MOST IMPORTANT DISCOVERY OF ALL**

Searching for the "Fountain of Youth" has become media fodder and yet the media has missed the most important discovery of all.

Isometric exercise makes elective aesthetic surgery for face lifts unnecessary.

CUTTING HEALTHY TISSUE

The business of "cosmetic procedures" has skyrocketed. Since 2000, there has been a substantial surge in elective aesthetic (cosmetic) surgery. In 2005, there were more than 10.2 million total cosmetic procedures performed in the United States. This is an increase of 11% from the previous year and these statistics clearly demonstrate that Americans, particularly women, are increasingly willing to invest in cutting healthy tissue to buy into the myth that enhancement means surgery.

> **FAIR AND BALANCED REPORTING COULD SAVE MONEY AND LIVES.**

In 1994 there were only 364,398 total cosmetic procedures performed; this means that the American economy propelled the aesthetic surgery industry to a gain of 2700% in less than twelve years. The media has sufficiently supported the newest, modern, up-to-date surgical, minimally invasive and cosmetic enhancement processes that taunt consumers into believing that anti-aging is all about spending huge sums of money while risking one's health. Fair and balanced reporting could save money and lives.

The upsurge in cosmetic overhaul demands has left no one out. More minorities are undergoing cosmetic procedures than ever; according to the American Society of Plastic Surgeons the number of surgical cosmetic procedures jumped 65% for African-Americans, Asians and Hispanics in 2006.

DANGEROUS AND TEMPORARY

New surgical procedures and injections usually have unknown consequences and even doctors hesitate to jump on the bandwagon quickly. Consider the quote from Dr. Kotler: "I certainly would not be one of the first to serve as a guinea pig for a new surgical procedure. I'm not sure if seven years is the appropriate waiting period, but there should certainly be a wait to see what problems develop over time in those who have the surgery," states clinical instructor Robert Kotler of UCLA medical school, and author of "The Essential Cosmetic Surgery Companion" (2005). "In the world of cosmetic procedures, it takes years before all the benefits, all the complications and dissatisfactions come to awareness" says Kotler.

Even with the new state-of-the-art minimal-incision face lifting techniques, there are still major drawbacks and serious consequences with every surgical procedure. "Even when successful, these procedures are by no means a 'permanent fix' as subsequent face lifts or other interventions usually are required," states Mark Berman, MD, Santa Monica, CA, past President of the California Academy of Cosmetic Surgeons. These subsequent visits for additional surgery, injections, liposuctions, peels and more eventually take a toll on the user's available income and long-term health issues can arise.

IS THERE A VIABLE SOLUTION THAT HAS ZERO RISKS AND NO SIDE EFFECTS?

The general public wants to know there is a proven, safe alternative to plastic surgery.

Facial muscles that are sagging can be retrained and lifted with resistance movements and the general public deserves to know that there is a proven, safe alternative to plastic surgery that will indeed lift, tone and tighten facial features.

> **ISOMETRIC EXERCISE MAKES ELECTIVE AESTHETIC SURGERY FOR FACE LIFTS UNNECESSARY.**

These carefully orchestrated facial exercises are not contortions. Rather, they are isometric and resistance exercises that address the cause of aging in faces. These specialized exercises shape and contour the face and neck muscles easily and simply without the high costs or risks typically associated with cosmetic or plastic surgery.

NEUROMUSCULAR FACIAL RETRAINING

The medical community has long used resistance exercise to correct certain orofacial maladies caused by injury or disease. Neuromuscular facial retraining, facial exercise, is the foundation of Orofacial Myology. This regimen has been used for years by physicians and practitioners whose patients have suffered facial paralysis, Bell's Palsy, traumatic injury and more to strengthen the facial musculature through exercise while normalizing the movements of the facial muscles with outstanding results.

Licia Paskay, Los Angeles based Certified Orofacial Myologist, trained to evaluate and treat facial muscle dysfunction, states, "Exercises for the face are very good, they balance the muscles and a balanced face makes a person look better".

> **I'VE SEEN THE RESULTS AND IT WORKS!**

According to Berman there are two reconstructive interventions (for facial aging): Surgical and non-surgical. "The non-surgical method is through regular exercise of facial muscles and this can be accomplished effectively without any of the health risks, expense, and pain or scarring of surgery or injections. I've seen the results and it works!"

Resistance exercise for the face works just like exercise using weights, body weight and strength training for the torso, legs, hips, and arms. Resistance movements for the face require the user to employ thumbs and fingers in strategic positions so that a contraction is caused in the muscles. Artificially anchoring one end of the muscle will produce a plumping effect when oxygenated blood is forced to the tissue. Dr. Berman, "Such physical exercise of the facial muscles can create a more youthful, healthier appearance by causing the facial skin to tighten up and become more toned."

Facial Exercise Makes Sense Medically

Most doctors agree that if you are out of shape you need exercise to strengthen the core muscles; it is absurd to think that facial muscles wouldn't benefit from highly specialized isometric exercise techniques.

Regarding facial exercise Dr. Berman states, "...this is a medically sound method of achieving and maintaining a more youthful facial appearance with the capacity of obtaining results that are comparable to those that can be achieved by surgical means. It makes sense medically. Like a face lift or fat injection, such physical exercise of the facial muscles can create a more youthful, healthier appearance by causing the facial skin to tighten up and become more toned. And it can accomplish this effectively without any of the health risk, expense, pain or scarring of surgery. Whether you're 30 or 70, you'll see a definite change".

> **It is absurd to think that facial muscles wouldn't benefit from highly specialized isometric exercise techniques.**

Most medical practitioners have not been trained in isometric facial exercise, nor have they had the opportunity to observe and witness the amazing results of resistance and contraction exercises. Because of this, they do not recommend these simple, non-surgical, non-invasive movements to their clients.

WILD WEST COWBOYS

Non-surgical cosmetic grade procedures are typically not covered by insurance companies. Offering the latest muscle paralyzing injection or those that fill and plump lines and wrinkles provides the doctor a revenue stream that doesn't require insurance filing or collecting hassles because the fees are paid in advance by those seeking treatment.

A strong stance against unethical, untrained "wild west cowboys" needs to be implemented by every state since medical doctors have begun to augment their incomes with injections and surgical procedures fueled by the increased demand for beauty and youthfulness. They are thinking more like entrepreneurs and less like benevolent healers.

Dr. Berry Lycka author of "Restoring Youth – How to Keep and Restore Natural Beauty" founded the Ethical Cosmetic Surgery Association to alert the public about the fact that tax cuts proposed by President Bush will drastically affect physicians. "Many physicians who previously offered services to Medicare patients will simply no longer be able to do so." Dr. Lycka goes on to say, "To provide income, many of these doctors will probably find their way into doing some sort of cosmetic surgery procedure. With Botox, lasers, and fillers perceived as easy to do, many doctors will migrate to these practices. To cosmetic patients it will be a case of 'let the buyer beware'. Many doctors are not adequately trained to provide these procedures."

Some plastic surgeons have created vehicles designed to educate the public while policing their colleagues' practices. John J. Corey MD, Executive Director of the Association for Plastic Surgery Awareness, APSA, says this website (www.APSA.org), was created to raise mainstream consumer's awareness and provide them the information, tools and resources for potential patients to research the background of a plastic surgeon before undergoing any surgical procedure.

THE RISKS ARE MORE THAN JUST MONETARY.

The elation of expectation, the fevered pitch of anticipation and the desire to rid oneself of aging facial features has prompted desperate people to act irresponsibly. Many go into debt, fly off to exotic islands and accept substandard surgery practices because they want to look younger. Health risks be damned! Hospital and clinic environments, no matter what country or hemisphere, increase one's risk of infection and MRSA, the nasty staph infection that can lead to death after surgery.

Before anyone considers a face lift or a cosmetic surgical procedure there is helpful information that one must consider:

- Each surgery involves 1 – 3 hours of actual procedure time.

- During pre-op the surgeon will use a marker to indicate the location and length of the planned incision lines. The patient is then given injections of Lidocaine and Epinephrine for pain and to prevent excessive bleeding.

- Choice of anesthesia: oral or intravenous sedatives will be administered. Even if oral sedation is chosen, an IV will be started to maintain the body's hydration level.

- Surgical procedure will likely include removing the tissue beneath the skin while either cutting or manipulating the muscle to create the desired look. The surgery may also include separating the skin and muscle from the skull to remove excess skin and fat. Muscles and skin are then sutured or stapled.

- During the recovery period the patient is moved to a recovery room to have vital statistics monitored for approximately two hours. Patients may experience sensations ranging from discomfort, disorientation, nausea, and change in body temperature which may cause shivering and sweating. Patients then may be given additional pain relievers and anti-nausea medication.

- Cost when combined with fees such as anesthesia can range from $3,000 - $35,000.

- Scarring and loss of sensation: no matter how nicely hidden away the scars are, cutting creates a loss of sensation.

- Weeks of bruising and swelling, infection, uneven suturing, and hematomas are some of the most frequent complaints and consequences registered with surgery.

Prevent Your Death

The most serious complication of cosmetic surgery is death. There have been deaths associated with cosmetic plastic surgery but the statistics are difficult to access because mandatory reporting of botched cosmetic procedures does not exist. This means that the actual number of deaths attributed to bungled operations is unknown and unreported because they sometimes occur weeks and months after the surgery.

UNTRAINED PRACTITIONERS

Medispas, situated in malls and other high traffic areas, offer an array of medical grade cosmetic treatments such as chemical peels, injections of Botox, electrostimulation and laser procedures. Most times these procedures are performed under the direction of a doctor, not necessarily a plastic surgeon or dermatologist, either by an aesthetician or registered nurse.

Be aware that any MD, gynecologist or even a dentist, can perform plastic surgery without extensive training or certification. It is a little known fact that hundreds of plastic surgery procedures are conducted each day in the U.S. by doctors whose medical background, experience or training is not board certified plastic surgery. Even more amazing is that this practice is not illegal in most states. It is increasingly difficult to separate the qualified surgeon from the unqualified quack.

The medical boards for many states do not have specific regulations for medical spas or their treatment menus so consumers beware!

THE BEST KEPT ANTI-AGING SECRET REVEALED - HOW FACIAL EXERCISE WORKS.

Specialized facial exercise techniques using only the thumbs and fingers can reshape and contour sagging, out of shape faces, transforming the features into a dramatically younger looking face. Without surgery, without drugs, without risk, without high costs, without scarring, without recovery time, without pain, without mutilation and repeat procedures, resistance training will provide a substantial benefit to sagging facial muscles.

> **FACIAL MUSCLES CAN ELONGATE UP TO 1/2 INCH BY AGE 55**

Gravity assures the lengthening of facial tissue - this includes muscles and skin. In the face skin attaches directly to the muscles. Over time the muscles and the skin begin to lose their tone and elasticity; this is when the face begins the look of age. Studies show that facial muscles can elongate up to 1/2 inch by age 55 and when this happens, the skin is dragged downward creating lines, creases and folds.

All muscles require exercise to maintain their form and shape. The facial muscles are no different - they also require exercise that goes beyond stimulation like massage or electric current or daily facial movements such as smiling, grimacing or singing. The facial muscles, like the body muscles, respond to exercise that uses both resistance and contraction. This action keeps facial muscles youthfully positioned because when muscles are stronger, sagging is minimized and the skin is tighter and toned.

Many facial muscles connect to bone only at one end; the other end attaches to skin or another muscle. This unique configuration of the muscles means that in order to sufficiently exercise a muscle so that it plumps up and lifts, an artificial anchor must be employed. This is accomplished by using the thumbs and fingers.

Sometimes those thumbs are inside the mouth while the fingers are lightly touching the face. It is recommended that the user wear light weight white cotton gloves while holding and anchoring facial muscles. These small muscles weave over and under each before attaching to skin or another muscle and that is why retraining facial muscles require that the user learn to isolate, anchor, then actively contract the muscle or muscle groups.

The many facial muscles and muscle groups under the skin respond well to isometric contraction. These contractions with resistance remarkably increase muscle tone and that plumping of the muscles results in a brighter face energized with increased oxygen; this is especially important for those middle aged and above who experience dull, lifeless skin due to a lack of oxygen to the outer tissues as a direct result of aging.

As the muscles respond to exercise, the face is enhanced as skin acts younger and muscles lift. The facial exerciser looks years younger as a result of increased muscle mass and thicker skin. Just as exercise works for the body, facial exercise works for the face and neck.

Sample Exercise:

Upper Eyes and Brows

Perform this exercise once a day, six days in a row.
Take one day off and continue for another six days.

1. Relax your eyebrow area and then place the three middle fingers of each hand directly under your eyebrows (figure 1).
2. Drop the palms of your hands flat against your face.
3. With the pads of your fingertips directly under your eyebrows, push your eyebrows upwards and slightly outwards (figure 2).
4. Hold your eyebrows in this position with your eyes open.
5. Slowly push your eyebrows down against your fingertips while holding your eyebrows high, and hold the contraction for five (5) seconds (figure 3).
6. Remove your hands from your face.
7. Breathe in deeply through your nose, and exhale through your nose.
8. Repeat the exercise again. This time hold the contraction for ten (10) seconds. At the seventh second, close your eyes, keeping your eyebrows held high.
9. Remove your hands from your face. Breathe in deeply through your nose, and exhale through your nose. Begin again, holding the contraction for ten (10) seconds and closing your eyes at the seventh second. Repeat the movement again so that you have exercised for a total of thirty-five (35) seconds.

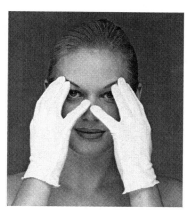

Figure 1

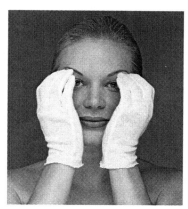

Figure 2

This exercise begins to "awaken" your forehead, concentrating on the area above your eyebrow to the hairline. Initially, you may see a line develop over your brow when you first perform this exercise - THIS IS TEMPORARY and a clear indication that your forehead has lost its firmness.

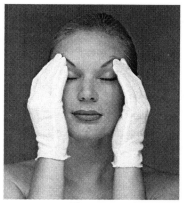

Figure 3

Anti Aging

Are You Fast-Tracking on Aging?

Are you fast tracking on the "Never ending desire for a more youthful appearance"? See how you fare when answering the following questions:

Have you begun using muscle paralyzing injections before the age of 40?

Have you had plastic surgery somewhere on your body?

Do you constantly berate yourself regarding your appearance?

If you have answered "yes" to any of these questions, you are battling with Mother Nature.

Trying to look younger using chemicals, surgery, and injecting foreign substances that have no long-term testing is detrimental to your good health. The medical profession that deals in enhancement cannot possibly predict how their patients are going to react to these substances or procedures over a twenty or thirty year span.

Once you've decided that surgery or injections is your chosen modality to look younger, you have set yourself up for failure. Why? Because one injection is never enough – twenty injections over 2-3 years won't be enough either and before you know it, ten years will have passed and your body is filled with toxic chemicals that may cause harm. And you still need more injections!

Same goes for surgery. Will one eye lift be enough? Will you constantly want to update your look using surgical techniques that contribute to an old looking face? Wait a minute you say! Isn't surgery supposed to make one look younger? Yes, that's the goal but more often than not, multiple surgeries make your face look like you've had multiple surgeries. The pulling and tweaking can produce a very freakish appearance, especially when fine lines and wrinkles are zapped by a laser.

The adage: "Aging Gracefully" has been replaced with carefully staged propaganda disguised as advertising in upscale magazines, TV and radio proclaiming that you need Botox, Restylane, and even surgery to look youthful.

This is a lie told by big companies who manufacture chemical and cadaver substances; the drug companies and the medical community have tons of money to sway your consciousness into believing this hype. They want you to become hooked on injections and surgery so they can continue to develop more and more substances for you to use. So what if there are deadly complications from over use?

"Over use" is big business and that is exactly what is hoped for no matter if too many injections equals repeat business. These repeat procedures equate to easy dollars for the medical community. And, there is little risk to them when they're using injections to line their pockets; no large insurance premiums are required for non-surgical procedures. That's one reason why Medi-Spas are prevalent in and adjacent to shopping malls and structures in high-traffic, high-dollar areas; there are no national standards in place to protect the consumer and they offer everything from facials to pharmaceutical injections and other medical procedures. The lure of the "lunch-time facial" with easy in and out can affect not only your appearance but your over-all health and well-being.

At some point, someone has to take a stand and say "Enough!" Taking control of your health means you must be willing to stop having frivolous surgery and multiple injections that paralyze and artificially plump up sagging facial features.

Taking back your power doesn't mean you have to look old or dowdy. In fact, if you stop squandering money on needless procedures Mother Nature never intended you to use, you can actually treat the cause of aging in the face.

Most aging is caused by loose and flabby facial muscles; if you're sporting a double chin, a wattle or hooded eyes, this is a result of muscles that are no longer strong and tight. If the apples in your cheeks sag even when you smile and your forehead droops into your upper eyes, do not be discouraged because you can actually exercise all the muscles in your face and neck. When you do this, your muscles will experience increased circulation, plumping the skin so that the face looks younger and fresher.

Using exercise techniques that are proven to lift and tone your face makes sense; there is no risk, it's very affordable and instead of looking freakish, you just look like you did 10-15 years ago...wholesome and recognizable.

Are Your Age Intervention Tactics Harmful?

Wrinkles on our faces and sagging skin can indeed provoke us to take extreme measures in hopes of stopping the dreaded look of old.

Men and women over the age of 25 have become targets for anti-aging products; we are inundated daily with slick, beautiful ads that point out apparent flaws like crow's feet, droopy features and dry, lined, parched skin.

Poring over glossy magazines and watching television ads suggest that our faces are in serious trouble unless we use injections, surgeries, lotions, potions and other expensive modalities.

Most skin care and certainly injections that plump and paralyze are laced with lab created chemicals but that may not matter to you if when you look into the mirror and see aging. At that moment you want something done and you want it now.

Playing around with injected chemicals sounds scary to me because there is always a risk involved using them.

Take Botox - it is a toxin so buyers beware! Small injected amounts probably won't produce immediate negative reactions other than swelling, redness, and tenderness.

Prescribed for forehead creases, crow's feet and other wrinkled areas caused by repetitive movements; Botox injections must be repeated every few months to insure that the muscles remain in a weakened state. Weakness in adjacent muscles has been reported as the toxin can spread inside the body.

There can be complications if you choose Botox. According to The New York Times, the FDA warns "that it also is probing reports of illnesses in people of all ages who used the drugs for a variety of conditions, including at least one hospitalization of a woman given Botox for forehead wrinkles." Uh oh.

Knowing that all drugs have side effects, there is a potential of experiencing symptoms related to botulism if you choose this drug. Slurred speech, muscle weakness and difficulty swallowing can occur. You should know that there have been spontaneous reports of death after treatment of botulinum toxin.

Fillers that plump are also quite popular. The lists of serums offered by Big Pharma grow year after year as scientists strive to provide doctors and their patients anti-aging fixes.

Some of these serums such as Bovine Collagen (from cow!) require an allergy test; other serums are deemed to be safe without prior testing.

There are two types of fillers: Permanent and Temporary.

Temporary dermal fillers currently in use:

- Radiesse - Radiesse is made of unique calcium-based microspheres that are suspended in a water-based gel and injected into the skin

- Hyaluronic acid - Juvederm - Bacteria proteins in a gel form

- Restylane (bacteria) - a biodegradable non-animal stabilized hyaluronic acid

- Perlane (bacteria)

- Hylaform (rooster combs)

- Sculptra (synthetic) - an injectable implant that contains microparticles of poly-L-lactic acid, a synthetic polymer

- Fat

- Collagen

Temporary fillers are absorbed by the body over time, some in 2-6 months and require repeated treatments to maintain the effect. Some fillers claim the effects last up to two years.

Silicone is the most frequently used permanent filler.

If these measures seem barbaric and very unnatural you would be right. Add surgery to the mix and all of a sudden, you realize that we Americans have become less than authentic. Cutting into perfectly healthy tissue, suturing, scarring, burning it with lasers and injecting chemicals can leave a person looking bizarre.

Procedures are risky. There are no guarantees that you will like the results. There are no guarantees that your health will not be harmed. There are no guarantees that people will recognize you.

Can we strive for natural measures to maintain youthfulness? Must we continually allow others to take control of our aging process using drugs and chemicals or do you believe a healthy lifestyle includes surgeries, injections and using chemically laden products?

Eating healthy foods, drinking purified water and regular exercise seems to appeal to most people. We know that these avenues promote good health.

Thankfully, exercise can stop an aging body and isometric facial exercise can stop an aging face.

Some people want you to believe that twists, contortions and scrunches are facial exercise. Well, they are not!

Facial exercise that tightens the features requires that you anchor the muscle or muscle group using your age erasers - your thumbs and fingers. The reason this is necessary is because facial muscles attach to bone on only one end; the other end of the muscle is attached either to skin or another muscle.

Anchoring provides the necessary component of resistance. Resistance and contraction of the muscles will cause these muscles to enjoy increased circulation which in turn provides them with new life. They plump up and support your skin so that you look younger, healthier and fresher.

The most impressive asset of facial exercise is that it is a natural method that works to change the shape and contour of your facial features. You need not be subjected to anything that hurts, or require drugs via injections or by mouth, there is no down-time or time away from home or work and most of all, there are no surprises.

You can look as young as you feel when you use facial exercise for your age intervention. Imagine yourself without hooded eyes, sagging cheeks and that dreaded wattle using only specific exercise movements to keep you looking good.

At Least I Have My Original Face

Now more than ever before – facial plastic surgery along with paralyzing and plumping injections have gripped the world. Frozen faces, overly inflated lips and the now familiar wind-tunnel-look has become a multi-billion dollar business with more and more teenage girls being lured into the trap as they watch their movie and TV idols morph into the senseless abyss of "cosmetic surgery."

According to a recent article, casting directors and other Hollywood types are not exactly thrilled with how their male and female stars have begun to rely on innumerable injections as well as nips and tucks. The celebrity faces are no longer easily recognizable and the actors certainly cannot emote or provide certain facial movements, expressions or characteristics when their faces are immobilized.

The popularity of high resolution, high definition television has caused major alarm for those in front of the camera. Scars are noticeable, Botox paralyzed foreheads look super unnatural and face lifts are definitely easy to spot. These so-called enhancements do not always produce the desired results of youthfulness; rather, the surgeries and the injections just make the viewer realize how desperate the acting community has become to look younger no matter how risky or preposterous the procedure.

Determining how a person's face is aging is easy and believe it or not, there is a non-surgical remedy that works better than surgery and injections. It is totally risk free, affordably priced and there is only one result: the user looks refreshed, younger and vibrant.

An aging face is all about sagging – sagging muscles and sagging skin. The medical community would love to have everyone believe that aging can only be stopped or remedied with plastic surgery or injections. This is not true.

Gravity continues to affect the muscles making them sag; no matter if you have had injections, surgery or laser, the downward slide of muscles and skin continue. That's why injections of Botox, Restylane, Collagen and others must be repeated regularly.

Same with surgery; if you have your upper eyes surgically altered, the downward slide of the forehead muscle will continue to depress the obicularis oculi muscles – the circular muscle surrounding each eye. After a few years, the same procedure will need to be repeated because surgery does not stop the cause of aging or sagging facial muscles.

Do not be fooled; it takes a lot of money to fuel cosmetic procedures. In addition to large outlays of cash that most insurance companies will not reimburse, there is the aspect of risk that must be addressed.

Every cosmetic procedure has an element of risk attached to it. Whether that risk is infection, pain, scarring, disappointment or financial, cosmetic procedures are not child's play. Frankly, choosing any injection or surgery should be the last resort.

Why cut into perfectly healthy skin when there is an all natural remedy to facial aging that is 100% natural and without risk?

That's right! Sagging facial skin and muscles can be remedied with isometric contraction and resistance exercises. These unique movements can reverse the signs of aging in faces and in just minutes a day using your thumbs and fingers your face can look younger.

Exercise technology for the face makes perfect sense. Just as exercising your body creates toned tightened muscles and skin, the very same principles can be applied to the face. Every area of the face and neck can be lifted and made to look younger without injections, drugs, risk or surgery.

Imagine your upper eyes lifting, nose to mouth folds flattening, jowls disappearing and that younger you becoming more visible day by day.

After a few weeks of exercise, you can turn to the camera (or mirror) and say, "All right, Mr. DeMille, I'm ready for my close-up!"

But Her Face

The average woman - the nationality does not matter - over the age of 40 is faced with a challenge like no other when it comes to her face.

That once youthful face after the age of forty can become a real health liability if plastic surgery and injections are chosen to cleverly disguise aging because most women who long to alter their appearance in hopes of looking younger forget that plastic surgery is indeed real surgery.

With the onslaught of certain television shows that portray only bits and pieces of what actually happens behind the scenes in a surgical suite or the segment is staged and carefully orchestrated to seem easy-breezy, the risks, a very real by-product of invasive procedures that tempt women and men worldwide, are not portrayed but artfully edited to only depict certain successes.

Bruises, discoloration, loss of sensation and swelling seem benign. But infection, blood clots, paralysis, brain damage and even death are very real concerns that are often overlooked and even played down. How about skin necrosis or puckers and dimples? These are very disappointing results that cannot be easily corrected.

We have all seen celebrities who have access to the very finest cosmetic surgeons who pay top dollar for their procedures yet they portray very dissatisfying results. Oversized, poorly placed breast implants, a nose that doesn't quite look right, a face lift that is pulled too tightly, injections that over plump and over paralyze features and eyelids that no longer close are common.

So, how does a woman preserve her face? How does she stave off the aging process without resorting to invasive, risky procedures?

Most women will head to the gym hoping to redistribute and contour their bodies but her face...well, it needs extra care.

There is a very simple yet specific exercise program designed to lift, strengthen and tone the face. Just as resistance exercise works for the body; resistance exercise can work for the face. Not contortions, twists or puckers that may cause additional woes, but a proven, reliable exercise program that works to reshape and contour a sagging face.

Exercising the face requires only a few minutes a day to execute the movements. You really do not have to wear special clothes or take time out of your day to go to a gym; a facial exercise regime requires only your thumbs and fingers in white cotton gloves.

Facial muscles are tiny; one end connects to bone in the hairline while the other end is attached to another muscle or it attaches directly into the skin. Special anchoring techniques will create a contraction in the muscle or muscle groups and the added resistance means that the muscle will positively respond by repositioning, lifting, tightening and toning.

Your facial skin is attached directly to the muscles so when the exercises are performed, beneficial oxygenated blood is forced throughout the tissues. This oxygenated blood works to improve the resiliency and appearance of the skin.

There is no doubt that sagging facial features make you look old. This look of old can easily rob you of your confidence; you may stop looking in the mirror, using lipstick and then you just might stop caring about your appearance altogether because it seems no matter what cosmetic product you buy or use, it is evident that nothing is working. The droopiness continues...

Topical products, no matter how expensive, whether they come from the drugstore, the department store or the doctor's office, cannot change the shape and contour of your facial features. Now maybe one day science will indeed discover a genome that will stop aging faces but until then the successful aging choices are very limited and most of them are risky.

Facial exercise can stop sagging eyelids, droopy cheeks, and even the dreaded wattle. Exercise is safe, it works quickly to lift the hanging features and the best part is that your friends, family and co-workers will notice there is something wonderfully different about your appearance. They will easily recognize you.

Most users believe that by using facial exercise one can look 5 - 10

- even 15 years younger in hardly any time at all using this all natural process. There are no drugs to take and there is no recovery time because you haven't undergone anything invasive, harmful or hurtful.

If you look in the mirror and see a version of you that resembles Great Aunt Hilda and you do not like what you see, you must ask yourself, 'What do I have to lose?' Only those sags and bags that make you look old.

Never again will anyone make remarks like "but her face."

Exercising Your Face - Fact or Fiction

You've looked in the mirror and have decided it's time to do something for your face. You're not exactly certain whether you should call the nearest plastic surgeon or take matters into your own hands. After all, this is your face and even though you don't want to look sixteen again, you do want to do something that will stop those tired eyes and droopy cheeks.

Facial exercise has been in and out of vogue for hundreds of years. There are many practitioners of facial manipulation; so what works best?

There's yoga for the face that aids lymphatic drainage, needle therapy via acupuncture, contortions and isometric/resistance training. All seem to have one goal and that is to help the user look youthful.

There are many benefits when exercise is used for the face: better posture is achieved as the neck muscles strengthen, a healthier face develops as blood flow is increased and collagen production is stimulated, and the facial skin becomes supple, refreshed and resilient. A facial exerciser will look younger as the sagging skin and supporting muscles reposition and align; the face will firm and lift.

Exercise is natural. It's not invasive, there is no risk and the only "tools" one needs are the fingers and thumbs.

Facial exercises using isometric and resistance type movements prove best. Why? Unlike other parts of the body, the facial muscles are connected to bone on one end only. The other end is connected to another muscle. In order to achieve a contraction in these muscles, special anchoring techniques are required for the specific muscle or muscle group. Just like exercising your arms or legs, when a contraction of the muscle is created, the muscles shorten and then "plump". When facial muscles contract this action lifts the skin because facial skin is attached directly to the muscles.

Looking younger is the mantra of most every baby boomer. This generation of "forever young" adults knows the importance of good eating habits, exercising the body and using the finest non-chemical skin care items. Facial exercise fits the bill for anyone wanting to look 10-15 years younger without spending their children's inheritance. Whether you're 35 or 70, you will see a difference when you exercise your face.

Facial Exercise –
It is Never Too Late to Begin

Exercise does a body good and the good news is that facial exercise can stop the look of aging in your face.

Exercise for the body has long been touted as one of the best ways to maintain your good health. It keeps your weight down, it revs up your metabolism so that digestion is better and it certainly can help to put the roses in your cheeks.

Without exercise your sedentary lifestyle can begin to wreak havoc on your heath as blood pressure readings may spike, weight gain will likely be inevitable and your once healthy eating habits may go bye-bye. This type of neglect sets up dis-ease that can inflict long-term harm on your health.

When you use exercise your body responds in numerous positive ways. Your muscles tone as muscle mass increases, your skin appreciates the enhanced oxygenated blood coursing throughout your tissues and an exercised body just looks and acts younger, healthier.

Many women who exercise regularly say that they wish their faces would match their bodies. After months, even years in the gym their bodies look youthful, sleek with improved posture and tone. Unfortunately, the exercise used for their torsos have not lifted or toned their faces and as a result she suffers from "Butter Face", as in her body looks great but her face...

Instead of seeing a toned, sculpted face, there can be noticeable sagging that detracts from a youthful body.

Eyes, cheeks and even the neck will begin to show signs of atrophy because aging in the face can become apparent by your early 30's. If you raise your eyebrows as part of your expression, you may have inadvertently created horizontal forehead lines. If you regularly knit your eyebrows in concentration, don't be surprised if you see elevens or double elevens etched firmly into your upper face. If you purse your lips, lines of expression will become evident around your mouth.

Stopping these types of expression can greatly enhance your appearance; most importantly, learning certain facial exercises will re-educate those tiny, hidden muscles and in time, the etching will become less apparent as the skin is better supported by strengthened underlying muscles.

What's really exciting about learning facial exercise is the transformation one readily sees when these techniques are regularly performed. Lifting, toning and tightening of the facial features quickly become apparent. Eyelids tighten, sagging cheeks lift and jowls and pouches smooth. Even the dreaded wattle can be reduced in just weeks.

Some people who have aging faces would like to believe that surgery and injections are the best route to stave off the look of old. The misconception is that these modalities are easy ways to remedy an aging face. Not everyone would agree.

Using surgery and injections require maintenance and upkeep. Consider this: by the time your face is 55 years old, the muscles will have elongated one-half inch due to gravity and disuse. Altering your face via invasive measures is not an exact science so the results of using invasive procedures requires a certain precision that is not always accommodated by surgery and injections that plump and paralyze.

This is why facial exercise, using your thumbs and fingers as your age erasers, is spot on with results that look normal and your friends and family will instantly recognize you. Using a natural, safe, no risk program alleviates all of the complications associated with aging.

Gone are hospital stays, time away from family, unnatural looking results, pain, risk, infection and more. Facial exercise deliberately begins to erase the look of stress and old from your face. Using these specialized techniques require that you spend only minutes each day performing the movements that lift, tone and tighten each feature.

Most facial exercise users proclaim that they look years younger and that results are evident almost immediately. Eyes, cheeks, forehead, crow's feet, lower mouth, neck, double chins are just a few areas that will benefit from a regimen of exercise.

What could be easier? It's never too late to pamper yourself or to give yourself permission to do something that is amazingly beneficial for your self confidence and self esteem. You will love your results, your friends and family will notice there is something wonderfully different about you and most of all, you will have learned how to take very good care of your face without one injection or a stitch.

Whether you're 30 or 70, you're going to see a definite change when you use facial exercise. It's never too late to look the best you can!

Facial Exercise and the Medical Community

The medical community concurs with Cynthia Rowland, facial exercises are an appropriate modality for treatment of many orofacial dysfunctions. Chances are almost every family will deal with either a stroke or other catastrophic muscle debilitating illness, trauma or injury – usually, this produces an inability to adequately formulate and articulate words and phrases. Most likely, these patients will require certain retraining from a speech pathologist or an orofacial myologist to strengthen the lips, tongue and facial muscles.

There are many conditions that can be treated with facial retraining; thumb suckers, those who experience swallowing problems, open bite and tongue protrusion can be successfully treated with orofacial myology therapies, orthodontics and other occupational modalities.

Orofacial therapy is primarily facial exercise that has been proven to alleviate the horrors of cosmetic surgical failures, aid orthodontic cases, Bells Palsy, Down Syndrome, and Facial Muscle Paralysis and so on. Facial exercise provides regained balanced symmetry to restore the face as it was before; this is very exciting information because in the past, what was done with surgery, can usually be accomplished with facial exercise.

One facial exercise client described how allergies had caused under eye puffiness and swelling; this caused him to look angry and tired. After just a few days of using certain facial exercise techniques, he wrote to say his breathing had dramatically improved and as a bonus, the swelling had decreased so he looked and felt better.

Facial exercise can also be used cosmetically. Rather than opt for a surgical procedure for treatment of a sagging face, facial exercise can provide much needed lifting, toning and strengthening of the face and neck. Exercise for the face produces the best possible facial appearance, altering facial expression in just minutes a day in the privacy of one's own home. The results can be startling and in fact, obtaining phenomenal results is very simple as the muscles rejuvenate and skin becomes revitalized with oxygenation. The stimulated cells thrive with increased activity that facial exercise provides.

Elective surgery is still risky as complications may arise; there's usually loss of feeling or sensation for quite some time after the procedure and sometimes the results may be disappointing. With exercise the muscles and skin lift, tone and tighten restoring the face. Most facial exercise users believe they look years younger than those who have had face lifts. In fact, facial exercisers look better and better while surgical recipients are thinking ..." when will I have to do this again?"

Facial muscle disorders that compromise appearance and function can be treated to provide the best possible facial appearance and better self-esteem for every user. Whether your need for facial exercise is medical or cosmetic, your face will enjoy the health benefits of rejuvenating, strength building movements.

Facial Exercise Defies Age Discrimination

Aging faces are everywhere and if you want to keep your job, maintain a positive earning power and remain confident in your appearance you might want to immediately begin a facial exercise regime.

It is the truth: Age discrimination is a fact of life in the corporate world.

The once handsome and debonair faces are drooping and that double chin is winning. The once beautiful face is amassing jowls and the resemblance to mother is developing.

This can be the poison pill in the corporate world because old faces can equate to old ideas. For more than twenty years psychologists and HR personnel studies demonstrate that appearance has a great deal to do with making more money and maintaining the status quo.

If you have experienced age discrimination, it's all about the face because no one looks at your knees and tells you you're too old, you may want to consider making simple lifestyle changes now before one or two incidents escalate into a serious matter.

There are only a few options when you don't like your face or your face does not support who you are:

- You can take your two or three week vacation, schedule a surgical procedure in hopes that by the time you are needed back at work, the healing of tissue and bruising will not be tell-tale evidence of your surgery.

• Fill your face with fillers to prop up lines and wrinkles and paralyze your forehead and the region around your eyes.

• Have strings inserted to temporarily hold up heavy cheeks and jowls.

Surgery and non-invasive procedures that involve injecting substances into your face, near your eyes and mouth may initially produce a younger looking face but you must ask yourself, "How many years do I have to do this?"

Is there sufficient testing of the substances to allay your fears of self-poisoning? What if these substances go the way of Vioxx, Rezulin or Seldane? These are only three of numerous drugs that have been removed after years of use when detrimental side-effects are known. This could indeed happen to injectable cosmetic fluids. Scary indeed. It is a fact that about half of new drugs are removed from the market or have significant warnings added to their labels within seven years of release.

The nip/tuck mentality has permeated the airwaves, slick publications and now the internet. Years past only those who were affected by accident or disease would consider having face work and that was in a medical capacity; now, even teenagers are targeted and marketed so they will adopt ideas into their psyche and words into their vocabulary that somehow makes it all okay for them to use plastic surgery and injections to alter themselves.

The irony is that even though surgeries and injections are on the rise, there are no guarantees that the procedures you choose will be successful. Even the most well-intentioned surgeries can go awry as evidenced at awfulplasticsurgery.com.

As a mature adult, looking healthier and younger is important and you do not have to risk your life to make it happen when you choose exercise over surgery and injections.

Consider this: Most plastic surgery procedures, including injections, will maybe shave off 5 to 10 years from your appearance. Each and every procedure is temporary so repeat procedures will be required. Pumping up your face with fillers and paralyzers year after year is an interesting concept and then supplementing with various surgical procedures may produce strange and freaky results.

That's why exercise is beneficial for every face because you know what the outcome will be – you will look like you – like you did ten to fifteen years ago.

Sagging facial muscles means droopy skin because the muscles no longer have any oomph to them. Exercise will oxygenate the muscles and that helps your skin to look younger and alive. Lifting is noticeable almost immediately as the skin and muscles are enhanced with exercise.

Using exercise is a natural and safe alternative to surgical procedures and the results will be better than expected as you see lifting, toning and tightening of your facial features.

Not just any exercise will do. It has been proven that isometric exercise is beneficial for the body. The action of tensing and releasing a muscle or muscle group strengthens them. Target specialized isometrics with resistance using the fingers and thumbs and the face begins to change as muscles reposition.

Imagine having a complete face lift using simple exercises that require only minutes a day. Every area of your face can look smoother and toned. Skin elasticity improves, your features are lifted and your skin glows with radiance.

Your confidence level soars as you feel and see that you look younger than your years. Trim your waist, lift your face, update your hair style and stay on top of your game for lasting success.

Facial Exercise Lifts Minority's Faces

Women of color want to look younger and they want to do it without risk!

In the last twenty years, extreme scarring, discoloration, loss of certain ethnic characteristics and high costs have kept Afro-Americans, Hispanics, Asians and other non-Caucasians from seeking plastic surgery but with the advent of improved suture techniques, new procedures and shows like "Extreme Makeover", more and more minorities are considering using cosmetic surgery to improve their appearance.

"The way plastic surgery statistics have escalated, especially among people of color, the trend to "look as young as you feel," has left no one out," declares anti-aging expert Cynthia Rowland, Los Angeles.

Statistics show a 65% increase in plastic surgery among ethnic groups over the past five years. According to Minority Nurse Magazine, "more Americans are getting face lifts and other types of cosmetic surgery these days, and more of those faces being lifted are likely to be non-Caucasian than ever before."

Clients/patients of every ethnic group use injections more frequently and with financing programs offered by clinics, spas and physicians, more middle income people are enticed by these lenient payment plans.

The top five surgical procedures most requested by women are liposuction, breast augmentation, eyelid surgery, nose jobs (rhinoplasty) and breast reduction. The top five non-surgical procedures most requested by women are Botox, laser hair removal, microdermabrasion, chemical peel and collagen injection.

All in all women account for over 85% of all cosmetic procedures.

Rowland explains, "There doesn't seem to be any area of the body that cannot be altered by surgery; your gender doesn't matter, what matters is how deep your pockets are. You're only limited by your imagination because surgeons and science are willing to go to great lengths to entice you to spend mega-dollars all in the name of improved appearances."

Rowland, a long-time proponent of "natural is best," declares that certain resistance type exercise will target sagging facial muscles so they lift and tone, giving the user the look of a face lift without risk, keloiding, scarring or losing your ethnic identity. Exercise can plump up wrinkle lines and lift sagging facial skin. Exercise can provide better results than a surgical face lift because it leaves the person looking like themselves, only younger.

Using Botox, Restylane and other fillers to prop up nose to mouth lines, sagging foreheads, droopy eye lids and thin lips are very temporary and costly remedies. These procedures must be repeated again and again to maintain the look of lifting and smoothness.

Facial exercise solves the problem of sagging by tightening and smoothing every area of the face and neck. The forehead, the eyes, the cheeks, the jowls and pouches, the turkey neck and wattle are all refined and lifted naturally without injections or anything invasive. Even the tip of the nose can be lifted! There is just no doubt that resistance training of the muscles can produce exceptional results that easily replace Botox, Restylane and most importantly, plastic surgery!

No risk, no pain, no scarring…no large out of pocket costs to reduce the signs of aging. This is a scar-less face lift that keeps you looking younger and healthier. Exercise is natural and the results can last indefinitely.

Imagine, exercising your face just as you exercise your body. See the results when you try this exercise: http://www.rejenuve.com/Facial-MagicSL.htm

Facial Neglect

Sagging faces and wrinkles concern just about everyone over the age of thirty. In fact, the search for the "fountain" has reached an all-time frenzy as consumers pay more and more money chasing after new, better and improved creams, toners and potions just hoping for a miracle in a jar that will erase, and then stop the wrinkles and sagging.

Sagging muscles in the face drag down the skin; you see the result of that when you witness nasal labia folds, jowls and pouches on the jaw and eyebrows that seem lower than usual. It has been reported that our facial muscles can elongate as much as one-half inch by age fifty-five. We certainly witness elongation in our arms, legs and buttocks; arms become flabby, inner thighs lose their firmness and the once firm derriere begins to slide into our upper thigh. The face loses its firmness, too. Aging isn't what it used to be but even when we slow the process with good nutrition and exercise, our faces show stress - and our age.

Here are five areas of the face that can make us look older than our years when muscles begin to lose their tone and the skin loses its resiliency:

FOREHEAD AND EYES

The forehead muscle, the frontalis, runs vertically from the hair line to the eyebrows. When this muscle atrophies, it elongates and adversely affects the eyebrows by adding gravitational weight causing the brows to lower and that's when horizontal lines develop on the forehead. This downward action also distresses the eyelids and they begin to show lines or folds and eyelids can become "hooded." Hooded eyes are very common; these heavy lids can impair your vision and make one look angry or tired.

The eyebrows sit on the top of the obicularis occuli muscle that encircles each eye. The obicularis occuli and frontalis muscles are muscles we use to "raise our eyebrows." When the forehead muscle atrophies, there is a noticeable reduction in the distance between the eyebrows and eyelashes. If you can't see your eye shadow, it's probably because the eyelid is sagging, wrinkling or folding.

Neck:

The platysma muscle in the neck is very large compared with the other muscles of the face; it runs from the upper chest area through the neck to the lower cheek area. When this large muscle atrophies, it sags quite noticeably, resulting in the dreaded turkey wattle, double chin and horizontal neck lines. The good news is that these muscles can easily be conditioned using resistance and the tongue.

Upper Cheeks and Lower Cheeks:

The upper cheek muscles, zygomaticus and levitors, anchor into the hairline but the other end of this 12-part muscle group inserts under the mouth muscle. When these heavy muscles lose their battle with gravity, the elongated muscles begin to "pool" into the muscles near the mouth and lower mouth areas, resulting in folds alongside the mouth, pouches and jowls, down-turned mouth corners and a less than re-fined jaw.

Aging faces have three choices:

1. Do nothing 2. Invasive procedure 3. Facial exercise

Just as exercise shapes and contours the body, exercise for the face can shape and contour the face. What happens when specific exercises are used for the face? The muscles become stronger and the skin becomes resilient; after a few weeks the facial muscles rehabilitate and the user looks refreshed because the droopy skin has been revitalized with oxygenated blood flowing to the tissues.

How does one choose a facial exercise program that will produce the best results? Resistance and isometric contractions reshape the body and these same principles will rehabilitate the face.

There has been controversy regarding the efficacy of facial exercises; the biggest misconception is thinking contorted grimaces produce the type of contraction that will lift, tighten and shorten the facial muscles. They don't. Excessive squinting and scrunching the face will contribute to further wrinkles and stretching of the skin.

In the face, the muscles are attached to bone on only one end; the other end inserts into another muscle or the skin. To achieve resistance the muscle and skin must be anchored. Only when the muscle is anchored can a resistance contraction occur and when this happens, the muscle responds by tightening and repositioning; the face looks younger because the muscles, just below the skin, are in much better physical condition.

Whether you are 30 or 70, you will see a difference using resistance/isometric facial training. Imagine looking five, ten, even fifteen years younger in just weeks.

From Drab to Fab Using Your Thumbs and Fingers

Many people avoid looking in the mirror. Why? Because their face does not portray the youthful look they would like to see.

How does this happen? Well, one story goes like this: A 55 year old woman was walking past a mirror and happened to glance into it as she muttered, "Who is that old woman?" It did not take but a few seconds for reality to set in - she realized who that old woman was.

She promised herself that she would no longer look at her image in the mirror until certain improvements were made. Days, weeks and months passed by and her confidence began to crumble as the image of old stuck in her mind.

Could this happen to you?

Our physical looks fade as we mature; our skin tone is different, our hair shows gray and our once beautiful faces begin to lose tone, vibrancy and radiance.

Surely you are one of those Baby Boomers or Gen Xers who wants to fight aging every step of the way so that you sizzle with enthusiasm no matter what your chronological age reveals.

You have probably heard that facial exercise can safely and easily transform an aging face into a more youthful visage but you may not know which type of exercise program provides the most benefit for a drab, sagging or droopy face.

Facial exercise that uses contortions, twists, puckers, frown, scowls and expressions that create wrinkles are to be avoided if you desire a younger looking face. These types of repetitive movements create wrinkles. Having more wrinkles is not advantageous if you want to look youthful.

Facial exercise that teaches you how to first anchor the muscle and then create a contraction will provide noticeable results almost immediately. Resistance and contraction assures you that those tiny, hidden muscles will take on a new and improved freshness as they better support the shape and contour of your face.

You may believe that learning a new exercise routine will be time consuming and difficult. This is not the case. Using only your thumbs and fingers while situated in front of your mirror you will easily learn positions and executions that require only thirty five seconds of your time.

Slow and deliberate contractions means that results are seen almost instantly, and as your muscles become stronger, results last longer. That sounds exciting, doesn't it?

This simple, natural method of facial exercise is superior to chemicals that are injected and facial exercise is more advanced than surgery. How? There is no cutting, there are no drugs to upset your inner balance and you never have to worry about not liking the results.

In addition, there is no risk of a nasty infection that delays healing, or scarring from deep wounds, no loss of sensation, or pain. The body understands exercise and it thrives; injections are foreign to the body and the outcome after numerous injections can destroy faces that only wanted to look prettier.

There is a plethora of anti-aging serums and potions, many types of injected materials available to plump and paralyze and surgeries for every facet of your face. Are they for you?

If you book an appointment with a physician that dispenses these services, you will be asked to read and sign consent forms that outline each possible contraindication. This protects the physician because the risks far outweigh the outcome but if you have complications, the physician will unlikely refund your money or schedule any free services for you.

When you choose facial exercise the promise is simple: follow directions, eat well, drink water and you will see results.

From drab to fab, facial exercise will have you looking younger, fresher, and more alive with skin that looks and feels substantially enhanced from increased oxygenated blood flowing throughout the tissues.

Now when you look in the mirror, you will definitely say "Well, hello gorgeous!"

Get Your Face Fit for the Holidays

Getting to Grandma's house is not exactly what it used to be. Remember the song, "Over the river and through the woods?" These days it is difficult to tell just who Granny is because she is no longer in the woods about how to make herself look younger; in fact, she looks pretty remarkable thanks to hair dye, trendy clothes and regular visits to her neighborhood Curves®.

There is one little flaw in Grandma's routine; she realizes her face is registering the look of "Grandma". That's right, resembling your Mother or Grandmother is eventually going to include you unless you become really hip about the fact that facial exercise can keep you looking younger.

Facial exercise that uses contraction and resistance will help you reclaim the face that you had years ago. Just like exercise works for your body, you can now apply the same principles to your facial muscles and they will respond by plumping up, filling out your skin and repositioning so you look younger and healthier.

If you take action now in less than six weeks your friends and family will see a visible difference in your appearance. You will know immediately upon beginning the regimen that your muscles are responding to this type of conditioning; you will feel the tightening and the lifting every time you perform the movements.

This means that cheek muscles will plump, your eyes will open, your forehead will feel tighter, your mouth muscles will become stronger so your lower mouth will not look jowly and your double chin will become less apparent. This and more as you take control of the return of youthfulness to your face and neck.

This is exciting news because you can save the money that you may have earmarked for surgery, injections and other beauty related expenditures; you know it is not about vanity but survival in a world that demands we look our best. We have had the information that old faces equate to old ideas for some time; we know that we feel more confident and happier when we see a fresh face looking back at us rather than an old, tired one that resembles you.

In just minutes a day, you can create subtle changes that will turn into lasting results. In the privacy of your home, using only your thumbs and fingers, you have the power to reshape and contour your face so that you look younger and younger without surgery, injections or risky procedures.

To help you get started today; click on the link to enjoy a free eyelift; this is a savings that equals at least $3500 to $5000 if you were to opt for surgery. No risk, no pain, no infection; only positive results.

Create that ageless face and you'll be the hippest Granny with the tightest face just in time for the Holiday season.

How to De-stress Your Face Using Simple Facial Exercises

Stress shows on faces. Sometimes it can look like a frown and sometimes stress makes us look tired, drawn, mad and upset. One thing for certain, when you allow stress to continually affect your face, you are destined for down-turned mouth corners and a perpetual scowl.

If you have been asked, "Are you mad at me?" or "Did I say something that upset you?" you know that your face is blatantly wearing your emotions because your smile has turned upside down.

You can easily remedy your facial appearance with facial exercise.

Skeptical? Probably.

As you sit at your computer take notice of your face posture.

Are you allowing concentration furrows to develop between your eyebrows? Does your mouth feel slack? Do your eyebrows feel heavy?

Aging faces soften because the muscles require certain movements to keep them taut. Conversation, singing, and laughing can help release tension but unfortunately droopy features will begin to become apparent as you advance in years. Couple that with tension from life's stresses and all of a sudden your face can look misshapen.

The old adage, "your face will stay that way" can become true. How we mold and hold our faces over a span of years and years attributes to the look that causes us to despair.

There is no reason to feel hopeless about your face. We want to look our best and we want to feel sensational about ourselves but sometimes we let stress, lines and a sagging face destroy our confidence. All this can be remedied when you spend just a few minutes a day being proactive with simple exercise movements.

Working from the inside to out your face can change from old, matronly even elderly to look brighter, firmer and certainly less stressed.

How does this happen? Exercise produces oxygenated blood to the muscles, the tissues and skin. This fortifies your face with circulation that pumps up the muscles and revitalizes the shape and contour of your features.

In addition to frown lines between the brows, a deeply lined forehead, a down turned mouth and maybe grooves, pouches, folds or jowls, and sagging muscles, facial exercise helps every area of your face and neck.

Facial exercise can help change the way you think and feel about your appearance. Using a dynamic approach produces a certain satisfaction that you are the master of your fate (face) and that you need not spend large amounts of money or endure certain risks to improve your appearance.

Using your thumbs, fingers and white cotton gloves one can easily begin to turn back the look of an aging face. Putting forth the effort works from the inside out. Learning then using isometric techniques involves anchoring, tensing and releasing the facial muscles. This action creates increased circulation so that your muscles and skin benefit from the oxygenated blood.

The stress and tension you feel and see in your face may be a career liability. So why not begin a facial exercise routine as a career investment so that stress and tension are alleviated in an all natural way. This means your face will no longer appear rigid and stiff.

The process is easy, it takes only a few minutes and in just days, you will see how the stress that plagues your face melts away. You will look healthier, happier and even younger as you retrain those tiny muscles hidden beneath your skin.

Is Yoga For The Face Really Yoga?

Contortions, puckers and grimaces are the basis of a new facial movement genre that is being touted as yoga for the face. Not only is this an insult to our common sense, it is easy to imagine that every yogi could be offended by these movements that produce lines and wrinkles.

Over the years snake oil salesmen have hoped their hype would result in a windfall of cash. They tout the latest and greatest cures with potions that no one has tested hoping that you, the hopeful, unsuspecting public, will buy into their spiel that will line their pockets with your hard earned dollars.

A well-respected magazine and a news leader recently reviewed these facial movements. There was no mention of results and there were no credible testimonials to accompany the information. What we did see were photos of facial contortions, puckers and grimaces.

These photos clearly demonstrate how wrinkles are formed. When you repetitively create lines and wrinkles with contortions and the like, it is possible that the face will begin to resemble that look. Think frown lines. If you have them it is because you have repetitively made that grimace over and over again.

The muscles and skin work together to create the look your face portrays; muscles that are strong support the skin...muscles that are lax allow the skin to wrinkle. Strong muscles plus energized skin equals a youthful appearance.

Using resistance with anchoring techniques is the only way to develop stronger facial muscles. Here's why: facial muscles attach to bone only on one end, the other end attaches to skin or another muscle. Without anchoring and resistance the muscles cannot achieve a contraction.

Consider this: open your mouth wide, now close it and open it three times. Sure you might feel a slight stirring in the lower face muscles but add resistance by placing the forefinger and the middle finger lightly on your bottom teeth. Open your mouth. Push your fingertips downward as you try to close your mouth. Aha! This is resistance you can definitely feel the muscles respond under your chin and up the sides of your face.

Without the resistance, the movement is merely a contortion. There is nothing significant that could truly change the shape and contour of your neck and face if you do not have resistance and contraction.

No matter what the marketing gimmick if you are hoping that a grimace, a pucker, a twist or a contortion is going to give you a younger looking face, you will be disappointed.

Talking, laughing, yelling at your kids, singing - the normal everyday activities will not stop muscles from elongating. It is the elongation of our facial muscles that produce that aged look.

Stopping the muscles from pooling as they head downward into other muscles requires action that is far greater than twists and puckers.

Our bodies experience slack muscles: our waists thicken, arms become flabby and our hips can change shape all because of atrophied muscles.

When you want to revamp your body, you head to the gym, drag out weights and hit the machines. You begin contracting those muscles using resistance.

The muscles in the body just like the muscles in the face will plump up and reposition when they are proficiently exercised. Without the resistance and contraction of the muscles, the body, like the face, will not receive the results you desire.

Anchoring helps isolate the facial muscles. Using your fingers and thumbs will create the needed resistance to lift a sagging forehead, heavy cheeks and even jowls and pouches. This type of facial exercise is the ultimate natural cosmetic enhancement because it can lift, tighten and tone droopy muscles and skin in hardly any time at all.

You know the risks and complications of surgery and invasive procedures but do you know that injecting foreign substances is risky, too? Looking younger in today's society has triggered an avalanche of new drugs, topical preparations, bizarre surgery techniques and even a resurgence of contortions first introduced in the 60's.

Be savvy. If you want your face to look and feel years younger safely without creating lines and wrinkles rely on isometric and resistance exercises that promote optimum results in an all natural way.

The process is easy and it only takes a few minutes a day in the privacy of your home to transform your tired, droopy face into one that is toned, tightened and lifted.

No puckers please!

Is Your Face a Couch Potato

The latest workout craze is Facial Fitness, according to Beth Teitell, Boston Herald newspaper writer and NPR commentator. "Your butt, it turns out, doesn't have the only cheeks that need exercise", she writes when interviewing Cynthia Rowland, facial fitness coach. Cynthia explains, "There are 55 muscles in your face and neck and they atrophy from disuse. If they don't get exercise, you are going to resemble your great-aunt Hilda."

Finally, fitness mania is now complete with the acceptance of facial exercise as a bone fide alternative to facial plastic surgery that helps every person over the age of 25 look years younger. It's about time, after all, for the face to be included in every exercise routine because the face has muscles just like the rest of the body.

Watch out, plastic surgeons! Cynthia Rowland is on a mission to make certain every man and woman knows their face can be saved with resistance exercises that will lift tone and tighten every area of the face.

We see aging in our faces when nasal labial folds develop between our nose and mouth or maybe it's a double chin that tells the world you're aging. Each area of the face can blatantly shout that Mother Nature is having her way with your good looks as sagging and droopiness become apparent in our faces. Imagine soft, flabby facial muscles becoming strong again as pouches, forehead lines and double chins are targeted and strengthened. When you tone and firm the facial muscles, the youthful contours of your face return so you look younger, healthier and fresher.

The facial muscles are structurally different than say the muscles in our arms and legs; those muscles are long and thick plus they're connected to bone on both ends. Muscles in the face connect to bone on one end so when exercising your face, you will need to create an artificial anchor, using your thumbs and fingers to achieve resistance. This slow and steady resistance will allow an isometric contraction to develop in the facial muscles so they lift, reshape and contour.

Resistance and isometric training are essential components to lift and tone the face with facial exercise. Not all facial exercise programs offer this type of specialized facial contouring; remember if there is no resistance, the movement is considered a contortion. These movements help your face to regain youthfulness and vitality so you appear healthier, less stressed and younger.

These specialized techniques are easy to learn and once you learn them, the technology is yours forever.

There are three likely choices when you see aging in your face:

1. Do nothing and let the forces of nature continue unabated.

2. Spend your children's inheritance on costly, painful and risky surgical procedures every few years that may or may not produce the desired effect.

3. Reclaim your natural youthful beauty with a proven facial exercise program!

If you answered yes to the question, "Is Your Face a Couch Potato" the solution is at your fingertips! Using just your thumbs, fingers and your white exercise gloves, your face will look like it did 10-15 years ago.

My Face Does Not Match My Body

Alas, you have spent weeks, months and even years sculpting your body with regular visits to the gym. You've invested time and money developing slimmer thighs, a tightened waist and a better looking derriere and then you realize something deeply profound: your face is the problem because it looks tired and old.

It is all about the face and it is sagging.

Sagging facial muscles can make one look old, matronly or elderly.

Just like the muscles in our arms, legs and body, the face is affected by gravity. It is also affected by disuse. This means that normal activity using hidden facial muscles such as talking, laughing, singing, yelling at your kids or your husband is not the type of activity that will keep your face looking young.

Using topical creams and preparations may keep your skin supple but by now you realize that your face needs more than topical treatments.

There are only a few options that will stop the look of aging. Most of them are frightfully temporary and they cost a lot of money.

Some health professionals want to inject the face with fillers that plump up fat depleted areas. It is not uncommon for a paralyzing injection to be used in conjunction with the fillers.

Imagine your face plumped and paralyzed. Will it be prettier and younger looking or will it look like it has been manipulated with drugs? The results cannot be predicted before the procedures begin which means you might look over-inflated, droopy or waxy.

In addition to fillers that plump and injections that paralyze, you may be offered expensive laser treatments or deep acid peels. These medical treatments sometimes go awry because they are performed by slightly trained professionals with very little practical experience. If you opt for this type of procedure, please ask the hard questions regarding training and experience.

Surgery is yet another option in the anti-aging business. This, too, can be a tricky proposition because it's expensive, temporary and it may not give you the results you desire. Risk of infection, loss of sensation or paralysis, heart attacks, and even death are to be considered when thinking of changing your appearance.

What do you desire? Is it the face you thought you had lost forever?

And, you probably wish you could have it without spending a lot of money to recapture it. Right?

Well, you can. You can actually perform specially designed exercises that will lift your face and help you get rid of that tired look that has permeated your facial features.

Sound too good to be true? It's true.

Using resistance with contraction movements, you can exercise your face in such a way that it responds by lifting, tightening and firming. This magical method will lift your eye brows and forehead, lift sagging cheeks and firm the lower mouth while sculpting a new chin line.

There's more. Your face will look refreshed and alive. You will feel better about yourself than you have in years because you are doing something very positive about your appearance.

You can learn these facial exercises at home, at your own pace. This is technology for a lifetime and you will not have to add anything else because your thumbs and fingers act as your age erasers.

Using your fingers and thumbs in white cotton gloves will change the shape and contour of your face. The routine requires only minutes a day and as the routine becomes familiar to you, you can zip through the exercises with confidence as you see your face respond.

Imagine, day by day, you see changes and in just weeks, you notice that your face looks healthier, lifted and toned. Now you can easily pass for someone years younger. Finally, your face matches your body.

The Magic of Facial Exercise

Once upon a time, a fair maiden met and married her long-time love. They had many children, lived in a beautiful home and enjoyed all of life's offerings.

One day as this mother, wife, lover of life, walked past a mirror, she caught a glimpse of herself and wondered, "Who is that 'old woman'?" After this rude jolt, she realized that her former beauty had begun to fade. What was happening to the face she had grown to love? How and when did the sagging begin? Was it blatantly apparent to everyone but her? Was there a way to find prettiness again? What were her options to regain a shapely, sculptured face?

Sadly, this "fairy tale" is repeated many times a day. The graying of America is a fact; while the Baby Boomers are turning 60, many men and women are endlessly searching for anti-aging solutions. They seek the latest and greatest remedy, choosing lotions and potions promising a "scientific breakthrough" just hoping that something will stop the tired, old look they are portraying. These aging boomers and zoomers want to look as young as they feel; rather they're faced with thinning hair, bodies that have become misshapen and faces that are less recognizable.

Certainly there are options. Pick up any magazine or newspaper, get online and you'll see plenty of compelling ads for plastic surgery, injections and treatments aimed at helping one look younger. Even if some or all of these methods are tried, the fact remains that aging gracefully is more than just "nips and tucks". Frankly, it's an inside job that starts with "the man in the mirror" and this is where the magic begins.

Face work in front of mirror is practiced by many models, singers, speakers and actors as they hone their craft for the audience and the camera. At first, you, like others, may feel uneasy as you steadily peer at yourself for a period of time; however, the mirror can be very revealing of who you really are and how you look to the world at large.

Here's how "Mirror Work" begins: Be alone. Close the door and move close to the mirror so you can intimately examine your face. Observe how you smile. Keep your face relaxed. How do you appear? Do you look angry or sad? Are your mouth corners down-turned? Can you determine what's changed in your appearance? Can you say "I love you and I forgive you" to that reflection looking back at you? Talking out loud to your mirror can subtly begin altering who you are, how you think about yourself and how much you can love yourself.

Facial exercise is one of the easiest ways to incorporate "Mirror Work" into a daily routine. That's right, exercise for your face is just as important as exercise for your body. When you are exercising your face on a regular basis, you are constantly observing your face in the mirror while you execute the movements to ensure that your finger and thumb placements are accurate.

As you spend more time gazing at your features, a certain type of acceptance begins to take hold in your psyche. Maybe you will begin to notice that you are more accepting of yourself and others, that little annoyances are indeed trivial and that you are becoming more becoming.

Yes, the magic of facial exercise works from the inside out, first making an important shift in the shape and contour of the muscles supporting your skin, but most importantly, there is magic when you shift your thinking to acceptance, love and peace of mind. There is magic as you understand that both physical and emotional change is possible. Like the song says, "If you want to make the world a better place, take a look at yourself and make a change."

Think You Look Like Your Mom?

Maybe when you look in the mirror you see a resemblance of your Mom looking back at you. You probably see more than just sagging or fullness under your eyes; you most likely see jowls, pouches, a downturned mouth, spongy skin, the dreaded wattle, sagging cheeks and more in the mirror.

These conditions - sagging facial features - make us look old and tired.

It is not unusual that a family resemblance is apparent because when aging strikes our faces we definitely have a tendency to remark that this must be hereditary because our Moms or even our Great Aunt Hilda wore the same look when they were a certain age.

Aging in our faces is sneaky; it seems that wrinkles, sags and bags can appear almost overnight. It is true. It is not uncommon for a wrinkle to seemingly appear out of thin air.

Seeing a new wrinkle upon arising may be a result of improper sleeping. These wrinkles that look so cute on a four year old when they awaken from a nap are surely disastrous when they are on the face of a forty year old. The realization that you have created this hideous crinkle may have you feeling hopeless and ready to succumb to the surgeon's knife.

Do not despair as there are natural remedies for aging that will not require recuperation or spending your children's inheritance.

Sleeping on a flat, mushy pillow can wreak havoc on your face, especially if you have a tendency to sleep mostly on your side. Same goes for those of you who sleep on your stomach. If you want to enjoy a wrinkle free face without under eye bags and sags, you might want to elevate the head of your bed by placing one inch thick books under the legs of your headboard while sleeping on a large, thick buckwheat pillow.

Bags and puffiness under your eyes can also indicate that you are using too much salt in your diet. Sodium seems to be hidden in many pre-packaged foods so if you awaken in the morning seeing puffiness you may have consumed salt laden goodies or eaten Chinese food or enjoyed certain vegetable beverages that are well known for their high sodium content.

Drinking water seems to have a positive effect on your face and especially your brain. Drinking purified water is a real boon to better health. According to the Mayo Clinic, water is a vital component to flush toxins, carry nutrients to our organs and provide needed energy to enjoy life. If you are short on water, your brain may act sluggish due to dehydration, you may feel dizzy and experience chills and even vomiting.

Exercise is another positive step that keeps you looking younger. The choices are wide and varied: walking, bicycling, Pilates, karate, Kung Fu, tennis, softball, volleyball, surfing, jogging, kick boxing, Jazzercise, weight training. According to Jackie Silver, author of 'Aging Backwards', "Exercise is the fountain of youth!" It is likely you agree.

Our bodies appreciate the rush of endorphins when we complete a strenuous workout. The sense of completion and satisfaction usually shows up on our faces as a beaming, broad smile. We feel euphoric...vital...young...until we look in the mirror and wish that our faces looked as young as we felt right now.

Alas, your face needs exercise just like your body does. Without it, the once vibrant muscles, the youthful, unlined facial skin is unavailable to you.

Even when you are meticulous and extremely careful about your face, including using the finest skin care, it is inevitable that your face will appear tired and elongated as your skin loses its firmness and its youthful contour. Exercise from the neck down isn't enough to sustain or maintain a youthful face.

A pro-active approach to a younger face is not about having surgery or injections; rather, a younger face is possible when you use facial exercise to stop the sagging and to maintain the uniqueness of your face.

Just as exercise changes the shape and contour of the body, specialized facial exercises, using your thumbs and fingers, will gently begin to soften stressed faces while lifting and toning the hidden muscles that support the skin. If the facial muscles are not exercised, the skin is continuously dragged downward by the elongation of the muscles.

This downward slide is what makes faces look old and that is when you see the resemblance of your mother, your aunts and others who are older than you.

If you are serious about learning the secret to a youthful face, begin a facial exercise program in earnest to lift, tone and tighten those sagging facial muscles.

What Many Doctors Do Not Know About Facial Exercise

Doctors know that their patients have muscles in their faces but when they think of exercise for the face to help their clients look younger, most docs believe that facial exercise consists of scrunches, twitches and puckers. They would be right! Most exercise programs are confusing and laughable; who in their right mind would believe that twitches and contortions would correct anything?

No wonder the medical community is confused about recommending facial exercise to their patients because the movements used by most of the facial exercise programs can indeed cause more wrinkling simply by accentuating the existing lines and wrinkles. Who needs that?

If one keys the phrase "facial exercise" into a search engine, depending on the day, one can easily find that over 1 million choices are offered touting facial exercise. When most of the sites are accessed, the reader can usually try an exercise proffered by the "expert" that promises to make the reader look younger. Some of these movements are quite bizarre; it is no wonder that physicians cannot legitimately recommend these exercises to their clients who want to look younger without surgery, injections or risk.

Carefully orchestrated facial exercises that use resistance training are indeed the most sought after exercise techniques because they truly address the cause of aging in faces. Some aging is caused by sun damage and exposure to the elements but the greatest cause of aging is really about sagging facial muscles.

Well-known cosmetic surgeon, Mark Berman, M.D., who practices in Santa Monica, California, believes that certain facial exercise can indeed produce younger looking faces as long as the exercise regimen is continued. He states, "I have seen the results and they're really quite impressive. And actually if you think about it, this makes sense medically. After all, when you exercise your body, you're going to tone and tighten the muscles in your body. So why not apply the same principles to your face. If you stay with the program, it should work indefinitely."

There are essentially two ways to change the shape and contour of the face; one is to alter it surgically, the other is more conventional, certainly safer and longer lasting and that is to bulk up or lift the muscles with exercise. Exercise will plump up the void created by loss of fat and collagen production.

If one chooses surgery to look younger, the procedure is not permanent and subsequent face lifts or other interventions are required to keep the patient looking young and fresh. Within months of a surgical procedure, the patient will notice gradual loosening and shifting of the muscles, reminding them that they spent thousands of dollars, risked their life with unneeded anesthesia, have a loss of sensation and scars that daily remind them of their choices.

The same continued expense is required if one chooses any of the injections currently available. These are expensive and must be repeated several times per year to maintain the status quo. But do they really keep the patient from aging? No. The muscles continue their downward slide so more and more injections are required. Ask yourself: How long can a person continue to inject foreign substances into their faces before they no longer resemble themselves?

Regular exercise of the facial muscles will make those muscles stronger and larger thereby causing them to expand and plump up. This action fills in the hollowness and makes the skin feel and look younger and thicker.

A regular routine of facial exercise will tone, lift and tighten your cheeks, jowls and chin helping you to look younger and vibrant with each passing day. Just think about it – you can save your money and take your new face on a well deserved vacation.

Why Facial Exercise Controls Aging

Double chins, softening jowls and pouches near your mouth indicate that your face is showing visible signs of aging and these areas will not improve unless you are willing to take control of the aging process.

Chances are if you are over the age of 35, you are beginning to notice slight sagging in certain areas of your face and neck; this probably has caused you to think about the remedies that are available to keep you looking younger.

Using injections is an option; however, injections are temporary, they cost a lot of money, the needles and serum inflict pain and they only work in a limited way. Plumping up nose to mouth lines when your chin is sagging or using muscle paralyzing toxins in your forehead when your eye lids are heavy is a complete waste of your resources.

Surgery can certainly hike up those eyebrows and provide the ever popular wind-tunnel look when loose skin is swept upward toward the ear. Never mind that dispensing with thousands of dollars, putting yourself at risk for complications and infection and settling for results that are less than perfect – surgery can certainly change your appearance. Surgery, too, is temporary because we continue to age. And, repeated surgeries can easily make one look freakish and unnatural.

The above options cannot compete with exercise.

Oh sure, the advertising agencies stake their reputations on brainwashing the consumer to make them believe that one can only look younger and prettier by enlisting the aid of a plastic surgeon who is willing to cut into perfectly healthy tissue in hopes that you will like the results.

Or that by making an appointment for injections of cadaver materials and toxins will somehow magically transform your tired, lined face into one ten years younger.

No matter that these injections can create additional wrinkles when the face is made to act unnaturally or that you might have adverse long-term reactions.

Exercise is natural and that means that your body stays safe. Using only your fingers and thumbs while wearing white cotton gloves, specialized movements can easily give sagging facial muscles new life and vitality. Just as you use exercise to keep your body sleek and toned, you can exercise your facial muscles.

Learning to artfully and successfully alter the shape and contour of your face when it is currently misshapen and spongy requires that you exercise only minutes a day. In the privacy of your home, you can take control of the aging process and make yourself look younger!

Sagging in the face, just like sagging in the body, is a result of muscle atrophy. Muscle atrophy is a result of disuse of the muscles; even though you have laughed, smiled, grimaced and frowned, these movements do not stop the muscles from elongation.

Gravity continually tugs at all our muscles – we see the result in our arms, thighs and buttocks; and, we see it in our faces. In fact, by the time our age is 55, the muscles in the face will have elongated about one-half inch.

When droopiness continues to affect your face, you will look older. Exercise that uses resistance with isometric contraction will stop the cause of sagging in the face and the look of youthfulness will return in just a few short weeks. Sagging cheeks will lift, the forehead will tighten, upper eyes will look vibrant and that double chin and wattle will be toned and lifted. Every area of your face and neck will experience the benefit of these remarkable exercise movements.

Imagine looking at least 10-15 years younger without surgery, drugs or risk. Just like exercise works to maintain the body's youthfulness, facial exercise will help you look and feel years younger.

Baby
Boomers

A Non-Surgical Anti-Aging Solution for Baby Boomers

Baby Boomers everywhere are searching for the Fountain of Youth and they have been looking in all the wrong places!

Men and women born between 1946 and 1964 are facing the most arduous and difficult challenge of their existence– the challenge of growing older while maintaining their youthful essence that stems from the Flower Power era.

The fitness craze that began with Jack LaLanne in the 60's has mushroomed to encompass many avenues and modalities of boomers seeking better biceps and rock hard abs. After years of working out, running, lifting, bicycling, tennis and more, these die-hard seekers of youth are still seeking something greater that will keep them looking younger than their years because their faces have not enjoyed the benefit of exercise. A toned, healthy looking body does not produce a toned, healthy looking face.

The crusade to look young has been lead by women; they embraced skin care products early on and they have continued to act as guinea pigs for the drug companies and plastic surgeons by allowing new products and procedures to be practiced and tested on them. Whether the procedure is strings embedded in the face, paralyzing injections or fillers; long term affects are unknown. The media's fascination with looking young has fueled women's desires making surgery and injections glamorized, sensationalized and well publicized.

The men have been slowly lured to join women into actively using skin care, hair dye and even plastic surgery. The metro-sexual males now frequent salons and spas on a regular basis for facials, hair removal techniques, massage and dermabrasion. Why? Who wants to look old and used-up? No one raised their hand.

This full-court push for youthfulness has no end in sight. More than ever we read statistics that demonstrate how millions and millions of dollars are spent each year trying to catch the elusive "young" gene. Some ads even suggest paying for these expensive, risky and temporary procedures with a second mortgage and maxed out credit cards; after all, with the average procedure nearing $25,000, not everyone has the kind of disposable income available that can buy a new face.

Facial plastic surgery is a temporary and very risky procedure. Plastic surgery requires frequent updating and even when the surgery goes well, the patient may not like what they see. Considering these surgical procedures are voluntary, it is frightening that people consent to them knowing that scarring and nerve damage occurs with every procedure. Blood clots, infection and irregular bleeding are also common side effects associated with surgery.

Injections, too, are temporary and made from chemicals that have no long-term test results. How many injections are too many? It is reported that patients sometime have more than one doctor injecting substances on a regular basis resulting in double the prescribed amounts recommended.

Facials do make the skin look cleaner and healthier but are you under the misconception that facials and chemical peels can correct a sagging double chin or heavy eyelids?

Plastic surgeries, facials, peels, or injections will not stop the root cause of aging.

The root cause of facial aging begins with sagging facial muscles. Yes, there is aging due to sun exposure; it typically begins to show up about the same time that your muscles are affected by the downward pull of gravity. This means that over time, your skin and facial features will be adversely affected resulting in the look of old.

That's right...as we mature we begin to resemble our mothers, fathers, grandparents, Aunt Hilda and Uncle Bernard. The facial muscles lose their tone and resiliency; in fact, by age 55, the muscles in your face may have already elongated by one-half inch. This means your face is sagging, pooling downward, making you look old and tired.

There is a solution. Sagging facial muscles can be remedied using specialized isometric contractions that work to plump up those small, wayward muscles. Muscles thrive when blood flow is increased – think of curling your arm using a dumbbell – after 5 to 8 reps, you feel the muscles respond. Couple the resistance with contraction and your face responds by lifting. In just minutes a day, you can pro-actively give yourself a youthful face just by exercising it.

The great part about using this type of exercise, rather than contortions, scrunches and puckers, is that these unique moves work for everyone. That's right, when the exercises are performed regularly, you will see a visible difference that is better looking than a surgical facelift. Your face will tighten and your skin will thicken.

It just makes sense. When you tone and sculpt your body with Pilates, weight and resistance training, you are proud of your new look. The same goes for your face. When you see and feel the lifting, your confidence soars!

Baby Boomers Are Turning 60

The 60's – flower children, hippies, tie dyed shirts, bandanas and free love. The Rolling Stones, Elvis, the Beatles and the notion they would never grow old began to permeate their thinking. Their new way of thinking made their parents shake their heads at a generation who embraced peace and declared to the world that they would stay young forever.

Baby Boomers begin turning 60! These bold, daring trailblazers have given "60" a new "look." Clothing, hair dye and vitamins have given the baby boomers an edge - Being 60 today is nothing like when their parents were 60.

This generation of new thinkers began an odyssey to dispel aging.

"Down with the establishment" is still their mantra today. An overwhelming percentage of Baby Boomers are turning to alternative methods to maintain and improve their health and well-being. Rather than medication, they've turned to meditation, acupuncture and exercise to keep them in better health.

Keeping Father Time at bay is truly a life-long commitment to a healthy lifestyle. We are bombarded daily with fumes, smog, and other air contaminants; lots of food causes gastronomical upsets and adds pounds to our physiques and our get-up and go has gotten up and left as our energy level plummets.

There are many components to consider for better health:

One of the healthiest things you can do to easily help your body feel more alive is begin drinking at least 6-10 glasses of filtered water per day. Water helps flush the toxins from your body, relieves most back pains and enhances cognitive abilities. Avoid drinking water with your meals so the digestive process can work more efficiently; try drinking a glass of water before each meal and then after an hour or so, drink another glass or two.

Exercise can prolong your life, aid in preserving your sanity and help you lose unwanted pounds. Resistance type exercise will sculpt your body and contour your muscles so it is a good idea to add weight training several times a week. Walking is a form of aerobic exercise that burns calories, improves your heart function and adds a boost to your attitude. There are many modalities of exercise from which to choose, find several that appeal to you and do them regularly. Just move!

Food is our fuel for our bodies. Consuming pure food in its raw, uncooked state— without preservatives or pre-packaging means better nutrition levels for the body. Eating raw or lightly steamed vegetables rather nuked or cooked, maintains the vitamin and nutritional content of food, adds fiber to our diet and helps the body alleviate disease. What about meat and fish? Animal based protein in the diet can be worrisome. Colin Campbell, a Professor of Nutritional Sciences at Cornell University and the senior science advisor to the American Institute for Cancer Research, says there is "a strong correlation between dietary protein intake and cancer of the breast, prostate, pancreas and colon."

Many nutritionists believe that 20-25 grams of protein a day is sufficient intake. Did you know that fruits and vegetables can provide protein? Yes, broccoli, spinach, carrots, cauliflower, certain lettuce, cucumbers, celery, along with bananas, peaches, cantaloupe and strawberries contain protein. We can completely satisfy our protein needs with fruits and vegetables. There are eight essential amino acids we need from food and we can get all of them just by eating nature's organic gifts.

Getting your zzzzzz's without sleep aids is a desire for millions of people. Many people feel they live in a pressure cooker and stress can takes its toll by disrupting sleep. A few nights of tossing and turning can affect our lives adversely. Over time the lack of good sleep could lead to health challenges. Sleep is the body's mechanism for restoration and strengthening the immune system. The goal of sleeping is to awake refreshed and revitalized. If you want better sleep you might want to take a warm bath before retiring, limit your exercise routine to the morning, avoid adult beverages and stop watching television from your bed.

There are four natural supplements that can help induce sleep: l-tryptophan, melatonin, valerian or kava. These are recommended by HSI Panelist Allan Spreen, M.D. Dr. Spreen: "If I really needed sleep (and couldn't get it) I'd never do any of the Rx drugs, period, but I would have no problem with proper use of any of those four (my favorite being l-tryptophan for younger ages, tryptophan or melatonin for the older folks)." Dr. Spreen also recommends Celestial Seasonings Sleepy Time Tea.

Anti-aging alternative avenues are becoming main stream. Certain "Rx drugs" have become suspect as many health practitioners claim that most drugs do not heal but rather mask the symptoms and even the FDA has come under scrutiny as drugs are approved, then disapproved when certain information comes to light.

Vitamins and supplements have long been touted as beneficial and their healing powers are legend. Supplementing your diet now with life-saving anti-oxidants will stave off premature aging, boost your immune system and limit free radical damage. What to take? Go to a reputable health food store and speak with their professionals; they will discuss your lifestyle, your needs and help you choose a beginning regimen. Take time to research trusted internet sites that offer information regarding your specific questions.

Life matters.

Boomers Want to Keep It Real –
Plastic Surgery Doesn't Cut It
Anymore

After perusing www.awfulplasticsurgery.com, it is no wonder why people are saying, "Enough already!"

Once you opt for a liquid or surgical facelift and that includes strings, your face will never be the same.

Oh you might be one of the lucky ones that resist infection, you might even like the new look that has been developed but one of these days, you will get real about these invasive, risky processes.

The reality of fading youth has begun to taint the senses.

For a while the sway, the lure of youthfulness was in our consciousness with entertainment television shows depicting desperate people clamoring to change their appearance.

Today we see air brushed models and photo-shopped celebrities that we admire taunting us with their flawless appearances in magazines. The lines of reality have been blurred as we watch our youth slip away.

Looking in the mirror only to see a less appealing version of ourselves is a shocker indeed. It is startling to discover jowls and pouches forming or a hooded eye developing. These tell-tale signs of aging can easily devastate our confidence and our self esteem.

Aging seems different today. Pro-aging, successful aging, anti-aging are topics discussed and discussed many, many times on a daily basis. Women, especially, visit and revisit their aging faces. The consensus is that they want to look the best they can.

The male Boomers', those fun loving hippies of the 60's, are turning 60 and they, too, want to look good. The question is: What is the happy balance that provides comfort and ease? Is it surgery or is it something else?

Looking your best can easily be achieved. There is process that does not include injecting paralyzing toxins or cutting perfectly healthy tissue. As one writer recently stated, "…most men and women of a certain age are satisfied to go gentle into that good night."

Exercise allows that to happen. Easily. Quickly. Naturally.

It is true, facial muscles can be retrained just like abdominal or arm muscles. Resistance exercise works for the body and for the face. Those hidden muscles that support your skin can be exercised in such a way that years can be dropped from the face almost immediately as features lift, stress melts away and lines smooth.

The bottom line is that we care about our appearance. We carefully choose our wardrobes, accessories, shoes, cars, products, food, relationships… our life is about our choices.

Surgery and other modalities of face-saving techniques never work in our favor yet exercise that uses resistance always works for every face.

Aging in the face is just like aging in the body; you can disguise flabby arms and thighs with clothing but how can one mask jowls, pouches, a double chin and more?

Creams and concealers will not hide the type of aging caused by sagging facial muscles, neither will make-up. The pro-active choice to disguise aging is facial exercise. It's natural, it's safe and there is no risk.

Exercise allows us to feel comfortable in our own skin. Surgery and injections may physically alter the face in such a way that even our closest friends may not easily recognize us. Saving your face from the inside out is seriously smart, saves you money and keeps you safe.

Facial exercise will change the way you think about your appearance as you witness subtle yet definite lifting, toning and sculpting that occurs on a daily basis. The movements are easy to learn and to execute them requires only a few minutes a day. The youthful results are long lasting.

No drugs, no surgery, no injections — it just makes sense.

So You Want To Look Younger – Every Boomer's Quest!

Here you are: A sensational woman living in what could be the most productive and most powerful time in your life. Your children are raised and you desire more. You bubble over with passion knowing that you have what it takes and then you look in the mirror and you are stopped, frozen, looking at a tired face that is drab and not too pretty.

All of a sudden confidence wanes and a rush of tiredness envelopes your body; this crushing blow happens frequently to men and women who are experiencing the initial onslaught of aging. Baby boomers have enjoyed maximum youthfulness; they exercise regularly, participate in spa treatments and facials, and wear trendy clothing with ease as they jet set here and there but their faces are telling their age.

Facial plastic surgery and the accompanying injections that paralyze and plump are being used at an insane level by men and women hoping to stop the tell-tale signs of aging in their faces. The drug companies and physicians have made consumers their puppets with slick advertising, air-brushed models and huge dollars invested in their campaigns to make you believe you need high cost, risky procedures to make you prettier, more handsome and prosperous.

In addition to surgery and injections, you have probably seen hand held electrical devices that promise to "give you the look of a facelift", alleviate wrinkles and perform other wonders in just minutes a day.

Television spokeswomen want you to believe that their good looks are indeed the result of using the device but do you know they frequently enjoy Botox and even surgeries? They shamelessly deceive the viewer, lulling them to purchase high dollar items while conveniently forgetting their latest visit to their plastic surgeon.

Surgery, injections and electro-stimulation devices are not quick fixes. Oh, it might seem that it's quick – you'll certainly look different when the bandages come off or the paralyzing injection takes effect – but you will quickly realize that there are other parts of your face that need attention. More surgery, more injections, more drugs, more risk, more outlay of cash and before you know it, your body is full of toxins and scars. Using surgery to look younger does not mean that aging has stopped. Facial muscles will continue to elongate pulling the skin down unnaturally while causing you to look distorted and older.

Pain, bruising, redness, swelling, loss of sensation are other aspects of these quick fixes. Every quick fix has a consequence; there is risk in every procedure that goes far beyond a little redness and swelling. Your body is never the same once you have allowed a procedure to be done.

What if you do not like the results of surgery? Does that mean you are willing to undergo another surgery to correct the unexpected result? That has happened to several people I know; botched eyelid surgery, lips hardened by concrete type fillers and implanted strings that create facial sagging are just a few ordinary mishaps. Multiple face lifts do harm long-term as prettiness gives way to that freakish, recognizable wind tunnel appearance.

Wouldn't it be wonderful to forego every surgical procedure, every type of injection and instead use a proven method of exercise to give yourself the look of a facelift? Does that sound too good to be true?

How would your face look if exercise lifted those tired, sagging areas like eyelids and double chins? What if exercise tightened droopy mouth corners and smoothed forehead lines? Would you feel satisfied looking ten to fifteen years younger in just weeks without spending a lot of money? Would your confidence return? Would you have more energy and passion about things that matter?

"Facial exercises may be good for mental health for the simple reason that if you look better, you feel better," says Newton, MA psychologist Laura Hart. One reason you feel much better is that you have saved yourself money and possible anguish by taking control of your face. "Using physical exercise can create a more youthful, healthier appearance by causing the facial skin to tighten up and become more toned," states Santa Monica physician, Mark Berman, MD.

You have exercised your body, now it is time to exercise your face using resistance and contractions, the very same movements you use to shape up your body. Facial muscle exercise results in tightened, stronger, toned facial muscles and this makes your skin look radiant, brighter and alive.

Imagine wearing a younger looking face that resembles 'the you' ten to fifteen years ago – your face is tight and lifted. Now when you confidently look in the mirror, you see a healthier, happier and certainly younger looking face. And you did it without risk, pain or spending your children's inheritance.

Beauty

Is Man-Made Beauty For You?

Growing old gracefully is passé. Rather than accepting those fine lines and wrinkles or drab gray hairs, many boomers and zoomers have decided to fight aging until they have gasped their last breath.

The question is: Has man-made beauty gone too far? Is the search for the Fountain all in vain? At the end of the day, is anyone satisfied with their face? Has the medicalization of beauty produced scary looking faces that have you concerned that you could be one of them?

Fighting the look of the aging face is a multi-billion dollar business and there are many components vying for the almighty dollar. The US plastic surgery industry claimed almost $10 billion in revenue last year while the US skin care and color cosmetic industry copped billions more.

Did you know that injections and surgeries, lotions and potions do not actually stop the cause of aging? Rather, skin care products, injectables, even surgeries must be repeated over and over again. Skin care and injected materials are absorbed into the body and then filtered through not only the liver but the kidneys as well.

The continued downward slide of sagging facial muscles may mean that a surgical face lift is in your future. This procedure will involve cutting healthy tissue and re-cutting again in less than ten years to maintain the look.

Does this mean that the face will forever be assaulted if one opts for looking younger for the rest of their life? I think so because big pharma is not going to stop creating synthetic substances for physicians to inject into faces. And surgeons, after all, cut and suture.

Page Six and other tabloids frequently portray actresses with their over-inflated lips and wind swept, no contour, surgically altered faces. Some tabloids even post laments and quotes from those actresses who rue the day they allowed someone to cut on their beautiful faces. "I'm hating that I did that to my mouth . . . I just want the mouth God gave me back. It was perfectly cute and I had nice big lips . . ."

Too late for her. Once a face is cut or injected it will never look the same.

Fooling around with your God given good looks has reached epidemic proportions and for celebrities, maybe surgery and injections seem like the logical solution to keep looking fit in front of the camera but extreme measures are not needed to maintain a youthful looking face.

Hidden facial muscles droop from disuse and gravity; this makes your face look misshapen, even old. In fact, when facial muscles lose their firmness, the downward sagging affects your skin as folds, creases, pouches and wrinkles form.

What works to keep your face, including upper eyes, jowls, pouches and more, in tip-top shape is a regime of facial exercise using resistance and contraction.

Sound too good to be true? Well, it is not. Just as exercise sculpts and reshapes arm, torso and leg muscles, the same type of exercise can contour and lift the face.

These exercises require the use of your fingers and thumbs in white cotton gloves that hold and anchor the very small facial muscles. The act of anchoring these muscles that attach to bone on one end allows a contraction to be made. This action plumps the muscles that support your skin so it drapes more naturally over your features.

Rest assured that isometric and contraction exercise will give you a younger looking face.

You only need to exercise a few minutes each day to achieve results and in just days, you will notice that your face looks refreshed, revitalized, tighter and younger.

Imagine the confidence you will feel when people notice your new face, the face you thought was gone forever and the satisfaction of knowing you did it yourself!

Facial Exercise is the Best Kept Anti-Aging Secret

Nasal labial folds: you know - the folds and lines (wrinkles) that are determined to develop into permanent grooves on the side of your mouth, in your cheeks and up to your nose. They're more than just laugh lines. Even if they were formed by laughing, you don't feel like laughing now because every time you see them, you know they are winning the war of aging.

Flabby muscles make you look older; if your arm muscles jiggle, those muscles need exercise. If your thighs look dimply or the skin on your upper inner thigh feels thickly soft, you can firm and tone that area with exercise. The same with a thick waist, a droopy backside or a bulging tummy; exercise is the solution.

An exercised body looks streamlined; improved posture means you no longer slouch and your tummy looks flatter because your core muscles have new life and strength; they're in better shape from oxygenated blood, contractions and resistance.

The face and neck muscles can become flabby, too. When these muscles soften and then droop, it is blatantly apparent that something unflattering is occurring.

Mind you, aging in the face is sinister because it takes a lot of years for faces to develop lines, folds and sags. By age forty, most people are seeing the early stages of muscle atrophy when their eyelids feel and look heavy, by fifty, the jaw feels spongy and you see that droopiness is affecting your good looks.

The look of old will affect your confidence and no matter how you wear your hair, or how much makeup you use, you will still see sagging. You can disguise a multitude of aging in the body by the clothes you wear – black, loose fitting clothing can conceal waist, tummy, hips, thighs and arms but how can you mask aging in the face?

Thankfully, there are safe and sane techniques that will save your face and they are easy to master. Facial exercises will quickly isolate the affected areas of your face and in just minutes a day, you can deliberately, systematically, and consistently help your face look healthier, prettier, and younger.

These exercises are not contortions; rather, they are isometric and resistance exercises that will shape and contour your face easily and simply without the high costs typically associated with cosmetic or plastic surgery.

From the moment you begin this incredible transformation process, you will see and feel the difference in your muscles and skin every time you perform the exercise movements.

Successfully exercising your cheeks to lift those laugh lines requires you to learn how to anchor the muscles near the nose so when they contract they reposition higher near the ear in the hairline. Have you stood in front of your mirror and pulled the hairline up and back just wishing you could iron out those lines that run from the nose to the mouth?

Exercise helps this to happen. Not just one exercise. Several exercises target specific muscles and muscle groups to contract the cheek muscles up and back to the ear. Contractions and resistance movements plump up the muscles, helps the skin to look healthier from the increased blood supply and gives your face a toned and tightened look.

The muscles in the face weave over and under each other; one end attaches to bone, the other end attaches to either skin or another muscle. This means that when the muscles begin their downward slide, they pool into other muscles and muscle groups, depressing the face making one look tired and even old.

You can stop this.

Surgeons do not want you to know that you can shape and contour your face with facial exercise. They want you to believe that you need injections, surgery and other costly modalities to keep you looking younger.

Exercise is so easy and it makes sense. Consider this, in just minutes a day you can create visible changes that will turn into lasting results. In the privacy of your home, using only your thumbs and fingers, you have the power to reshape and contour your face so that you look younger and healthier without surgery, injections or risky procedures.

For the rest of your life, this exercise program will work for you and you can forever look substantially younger. It's the best kept secret!

Try the following exercise for a few days and see your forehead smooth and your eyes lift: http://www.rejenuve.com/FacialMagicSL.htm

The Changing Face of Beauty

Not long ago, in the previous century/millennium, women and men aged gracefully. They proudly accepted the fate of their faces; no one was bothered by wrinkles, crevices or even gray hair.

The flower children are surely to blame. Those hippies of yesteryear firmly believed that they would always look like they did when they were swinging through the 60's, 70's and 80's.

It was when the drug companies formed an alliance with opportunistic physicians did they realize how desperately people clung to their youthful appearance. They began to formulate lotions and potions, injections that plump and paralyze and other modalities that would prop up aging faces and satisfy the longing caused by a nation preoccupied with looking young.

These temporary courses of treatment were soon accepted by the masses. In fact, the desired effect of just looking in the mirror became painful if the visage looking back was beginning to show signs of aging.

Spending after tax dollars to chase the youth factor has kept Big Pharma in the research and development business because they want to hook you into believing that you are not pretty or handsome if you are not using their products.

Celebrities were the first to use most every concoction distributed. It was and still is easy to spot those television and film stars who use fillers and paralyzing injections. Even though producers and directors might cringe because the scene lacks believability when emotions are thwarted if the face does not naturally respond, it does not stop the men and women on our screens from using these items.

The same goes for surgical procedures. These users of surgery and injections would like you to believe that that they look years younger because Mother Nature has been so very kind to them.

John Q. Public needs to know that fooling with your good looks can have dire consequences and that there is no need to go into debt or spend thousands of dollars needlessly on something that must be repeated and repeated year after year.

Consequences are increasing now that MRSA (Methicillin-resistant Staphylococcus aureus) has reared its ugly head. These super strains of bacteria and infection produce grave health concerns.

The administration of anesthesia can also create unwanted side effects; couple that with risky procedures and you have the recipe for disaster - The Perfect Storm!

Every procedure, every injection is risky.

Cutting perfectly healthy tissue, re-draping the skin and suturing it back together should be thoroughly considered as a life-threatening event.

Allowing anyone to inject your body, your face with serums that have not been fully tested or explored is ludicrous. Most injections used by the medical community have not had extensive testing to show results for long-term use. You are pretty much on your own insofar as long term use is concerned.

Perhaps you are thinking there is no hope for your aging face. Well, there is and it doesn't involve anything that would cause harm, disfigurement or risk.

Treating the cause of an aging face begins and ends with exercise.

If you are wearing a droopy, sagging face, it is because the muscles that support the skin are no longer taut. Instead they are headed south because they lack exercise. Exercise for the face will plump up the muscles, force oxygenate blood to the tissues and help you look years younger when you dedicate only a few minutes per day to a routine.

Do not believe for one minute that surgery or injections will work faster, better, longer than facial exercise. They will not. Just because sutures have been removed and the suture line looks less red than it did initially, does not mean you are healed from an invasive procedure. It takes months and months, maybe even a year or more for complete healing to occur.

If you erroneously believe that those paralyzing and plumping injections have stopped the aging process, think again. Aging continues to affect the downward slide of your facial muscles even if they are propped up and paralyzed.

As the old adage says, "You cannot fool Mother Nature." Be safe, exercise your face and look recognizable for many years to come.

Women Dying To Look Beautiful

Another young, vibrant woman died in late September during a recent liposuction procedure in Toronto. How sad that this talented, successful, single mother lost her life hoping to rid her tummy of a little mound of fat.

It is most bizarre that her surgeon had no specialties and no hospital privileges. She, the surgeon, was training in family medicine but she is not listed as an accredited family practitioner with the College of Family Physicians of Canada.

The scenario of allowing untrained and unqualified practitioners to call themselves cosmetic surgeons that actually perform surgeries is repeated many times a day in many areas of the world.

In the US plastic surgeons must undergo licensing and adhere to strict regulations, but there's little to stop general practitioners from calling themselves cosmetic surgeons and performing the same procedures that licensed plastic surgeons perform.

Family doctors, physicians, not trained in plastic surgery are performing cosmetic procedures because injections that plump and paralyze, liposuction, surgery and other procedures are very, very lucrative to their bottom line. They are in it for the money.

This is a growing public health risk and lax standards permitted this death to happen. It is vitally important to your health and well being to scrutinize the qualifications and training of a practitioner if you are considering any invasive procedures. This absolutely includes injections as well as surgery because injections are invasive.

Do not be intimidated or flustered to ask when, where and how extensive the doctor has been trained in any procedure. Some physicians are trained only hours over a weekend in certain procedures. You must remember that cosmetic surgeon is a misnomer, there really isn't such a distinction in the medical community.

Oh sure there are physicians who call themselves cosmetic surgeons but their training may have been in dentistry, internal medicine or proctology. In other words you really need to think carefully about allowing anyone the opportunity to fool with your long-term health and well-being.

This includes physicians who are practicing in foreign countries. There have been incidents of botched procedures and even deaths directly attributed to untrained and unlicensed, unscrupulous people vying for your dollar. They seem to smell desperation like sharks swimming after blood. Shame on you if you fall for their under-handed ploys. You must perform your due diligence and ask the hard questions before you consider booking your travel or their services.

Liposuction, breast augmentation, brow lifts, facelifts, injections and more lure unsuspecting aging men and women into believing that nothing untoward could ever happen to them.

The statistics of procedures that have been botched or resulted in death are not easily obtained. This is not surprising when you consider how long the industry has gone unregulated. These are toxic secrets that have been hidden from view for a very long time.

There are reported deaths in 2007 from Arizona. The circumstances are so bizarre but you must know how people parade themselves as surgeons when they are not. The Arizona Republic reports on July 12, that a massage therapist performed a liposuction procedure in which a woman died.

A homeopathic physician who was denied a medical doctor's license by the state board did another procedure in which a patient died. Others who performed cosmetic surgery did not have formal medical training; include a bookkeeper and a former restaurant owner. Egads!

Cardiac arrest, respiratory arrest, stroke, paralysis, blood clots, adverse reactions to anesthesia, unqualified and untrained personnel are serious complications that most likely can be avoided if you wisely understand that fooling with Mother Nature's handiwork can have dire consequences.

What about those shysters who inject fake serums into their unsuspecting clients? This was reported in Florida when four people went into a coma after receiving botulism and again in Las Vegas when a doc and his wife knowingly injected patients with botulism toxin type A - a cheaper form of Botox®. In Queens, NY, a beautician was arrested after administering fake cosmetic injections into her spa patients.

These and other sad stories are repeated many times during a year. No one intends to become a statistic and there is only one, sure-fire way to make certain you remain safe: Rely on facial exercise to maintain a youthful face.

Botox

Beauty Cannot Be Found At the Tip of A Syringe

It's a hard lesson to learn but beauty just cannot be found at the end of a scalpel or the tip of a syringe. The only fountain of youth that is guaranteed to keep your face looking younger is facial exercise.

Injections using serums that paralyze and plump may in time have a negative effect on faces because these injections do nothing to stop the aging process. If one stops using injectable drugs the face may look distorted and droopier than it was before the injections began.

Repeated injections may produce different results each time and they may not always look pleasing. It's like going to your hairdresser; sometimes the cut and style is absolutely perfect and then the next two times, it's just a little off.

Remember, these upscale purchases buy risks and complications. These can include excessive bruising and blurred vision; sometimes your smile can be negatively affected, or you may experience only an overly dry mouth. Drugs can have adverse effects.

Surgery and injections are temporary. If you decide to repeat certain facial surgeries, you may look warped after the third or fourth procedure. And, have you noticed that certain people begin to resemble each other? Think "the Joker" from Batman.

Let me remind you that surgery is forever so once your healthy tissue is cut and sutured, you never really look like you again.

Some people mistakenly believe that surgery and injections are the quick fixes – they are not! Recovery poses situations like time away from family, possible infection, pain, swelling, bruising and excessive bleeding.

Common sense dictates that fooling with your God-given good looks may result in disastrous consequences.

Why not play it smart and use exercise to look younger?

None of the above conditions are present when one chooses exercise. Exercise is natural, the movements require only a few minutes each day and your face begins to return to a more youthful look in hardly anytime at all.

You are probably curious how exercise can help you look like you did five, ten, even fifteen years ago. The process is simple.

First of all, a face looks aged when the muscles hidden beneath the skin begin to lose their tone. When this happens, the muscles elongate and this action then drags down the skin. The muscles pool into other muscles and muscle groups resulting in the formation of wrinkles and excessive sagging.

If you have hooded eyes, jowls, pouches or even a turkey neck, this is a direct result of lax muscle tone and these conditions can be remedied with facial exercise.

Just as your body responds to resistant exercise, your tiny facial muscles can benefit from isometric contractions that reposition the muscles more youthfully. The facial skin is attached to the muscles and when you exercise your face, you increase the circulation and that aids in developing younger looking skin.

From the inside out, recapture the face you thought was lost forever.

Using your thumbs and fingers in white cotton gloves you will soon understand how resistance and contraction plumps up your facial muscles that are sagging from atrophy.

The plumping happens quickly as oxygenated blood is forced to the tissues. The skin looks healthier, your face is tighter and you look younger.

Will you look like you are twenty again? Of course not but your face will look more toned, tightened and lifted as a result of exercise.

The beauty of learning an effective exercise routine for your face is that once you have learned the techniques, you have this technology for life.

This means you will always look substantially younger than your peers who have not exercised their faces.

Your confidence level will soar when you look in the mirror and see a lifted, toned and tightened face smiling back at you. This is your time to think about your looks and you can outshine any celebrity with your beautiful exercised face.

Botox - Wrinkles and Job Insecurity

Botox, once the "darling" of the celebrity crowd has moved front and center into the business world where daring men and women go to great lengths to disguise frown lines, age lines and anything resembling Mother Nature's wicked march across their faces.

Why? They know their jobs require them to look fresh and healthy; old, deeply lined, tired, faces are becoming passé because ideas coming from someone wearing an out of shape, soft, sagging face can equate to old, stale ideas in the business arena. Botox, once used primarily by women is now used by more and more men as they, too, realize the importance of maintaining a more youthful appearance. Their jobs may just depend on it.

Some say Botox is a wonder drug that smoothes wrinkles and indeed it does; however there are a few drawbacks that are a concern. According to the Independent, a London based newspaper, "Increasingly, people who have used or considered Botox are worried about possible side-effects, including developing fresh wrinkles as they change expressions to compensate for the paralysis in parts of their faces."

Wait! Develop fresh wrinkles??? Dr. David Becker, professor of dermatology, Cornell Medical College, issued a caution linking Botox injections to development of new wrinkles when users recreate facial expressions. The paralyzed muscles cannot respond so nearby muscles are automatically summoned. The result? New wrinkles. Oh dear.

Botox has been used since the early 1990's to treat lines and wrinkles associated with the motion of underlying facial muscles. Expressions such as excessive brow movements can cause horizontal lines, eye squints produce crows feet and subtle sagging of the facial muscles can make skin drape strangely.

Botox cannot stop the sagging muscles; in fact, Dr Michelle Copeland, a plastic surgeon in NY said, "...Because Botox wears off, more frequent injections are required to maintain its effects or the patient's face will return to its wrinkly state."

And what if you are wearing a "severe/angry facial expression" that after botox develops into a frozen, smooth, plastic look? Does that work to your advantage? Perhaps. Your facial expressions are who you are; take those away and you just may resemble a Stepford wife; however, there are those users who swear that having a subdued expression has helped them with intense negotiations and other business related circumstances, calling the poker faced look a "competitive edge."

Just remember:

1) Botox can result in the development of fine lines and wrinkles in other areas of the face. 2) Botox requires more painful injections to maintain results. 3) Botox is costly; treatments range from $200-$600. 4) Botox can result in undesirable side effects including allergic reactions, difficulty breathing, unusual muscle weakness, chest pain, headaches and dizziness.

What if you could avoid needles and scalpels and look younger? What if you could be in charge of the aging process and look healthier? What if you could manipulate and retrain your facial muscles to look and act younger without resorting to expensive, barbaric measures that are risky and dangerous? Well, you can!

Muscles in the face can be retrained when they are exercised. Your forehead muscle can tighten, crows feet can diminish and your face can look firm and healthy without any risk from costly injections or fillers. And actually if you think about it, facial exercise makes sense medically. After all, when you exercise your body, you're going to tone and tighten the muscles in your body. So why not apply the same principles to your face? If you continue to exercise your face, you will look substantially younger indefinitely.

Could Botox Create The Zombie Nation?

Looking your best has never been easier. There are so many avenues from which to choose - just thumb through any slick magazine, your local newspaper or log on to a favorite news site and the choices become practically endless because many, many advertisers are vying for your dollars proclaiming that wrinkles, sags and bags can be remedied using these expensive lotions, potions and serums.

Buying good looks is very common. No matter if you are a boardroom executive or a bored housewife, you have probably given some thought to creating a better looking face. After all, Mother Nature isn't always kind to faces over forty.

Looking younger is an international epidemic resulting from the idea that we are living longer than our ancestors and that if we want to successfully compete in today's world we must continue to look young and vibrant.

Again and again we have heard that sixty is the new forty; we know that our grandparents and parents did not look like we look now at the same age and most of us have decided that we are going to fight aging every step of the way.

There is nothing wrong with fighting a good fight to keep an aged face at bay, after all, who wants to look old? It's the methods offered that can cause great concern for our long-term good health that needs to get and keep our attention.

Maybe you have decided that plastic surgery is not for you. Cutting perfectly healthy tissue in the name of beauty has its drawbacks - the incidence of infection, recovery time, time away from the family and job, dissatisfaction with the results and the risk of death are all hazards that can be avoided just by saying no.

What about a "liquid facelift"? It isn't so dangerous, right?

A liquid facelift is performed with needles bearing serums that plump and paralyze. It seems that users of these serums have forgotten or maybe they have never been told that long-term testing has not been completed on most of these toxic injectables, so it's truly a buyer beware life and death scenario.

What is really interesting about these serums is the paperwork presented by physicians that require your signature when you are serious about using these preparations.

Usually one believes that a physician has your best interests at heart but after reading the paperwork that outlines the contraindications of Botox, one has to step back and consider the blatant ramifications of allowing a toxin to be willingly injected into the body.

Knowing that Botox has only been approved for the frown lines between the eye brows, it is curious that it is being used "off label" for other areas such as crow's feet, vertical neck bands and more.

The warnings include the usual superfluous ones like swelling, redness at the injection site and maybe a drooping eyelid that will probably correct itself in a few weeks - certainly in less than three months. The very telling danger lies in the words of caution such as:

- Paralysis of a nearby muscle that could interfere with opening the eye(s)

- Disorientation, double vision or past pointing (dizziness or imbalance)

- Temporary asymmetrical appearance

- Abnormal or lack of facial expression

- Local numbness

- Headache, nausea or flu-like symptoms

- Swallowing, speech or respiratory disorders

- Facial pain

- Product ineffectiveness

- Muscle atrophy

- Nerve irritability

- Production of antibodies with unknown effect to general health

- Death

- Serious disability

Some of the most unusual authorization aspects are the statements that a patient must agree to if they choose Botox:

- I am aware and accept that no guarantees about the results of the procedure have been made or implied.

- I understand and accept that the long-term effects of repeated use of Botox Cosmetic are as yet unknown.

The effects of Botox are temporary yet the effects can be lethal.

Scary indeed especially now that there is evidence that the serum migrates via the nerve cells. Having a Botox'd brain may mean you no longer have full access to your faculties. What if this results in slowed or deliberate speech or even worse?

Why chance any occurrence that could potentially harm your good health? What price beauty indeed?

What if you could easily begin to stop frown lines without using anything harmful? Would you be interested in knowing that a tightened forehead is possible using only exercise? Could you invest in yourself with an all-natural alternative that requires no doctor visits or any type of invasive procedure?

This all-natural alternative is isometric and resistance exercise. Yes! Exercise can easily change the shape and contour of your face and once you learn the routine, there is no need for further expenditure because the technology is yours forever. Just keep in mind that exercise can work for you like facial plastic surgery and Botox by addressing: droopy eyelids and brows, sagging cheeks, jowls, pouches, double chins and more.

Imagine looking ten to fifteen years younger without ever relying on invasive injections in the face or risky surgeries that require repeating. These modalities do not always make you look younger; rather surgery and injections mostly make you look like you have had work done and maybe even a little freakish.

Facial Exercise is the Best Investment For Long Term Beauty

Imagine taking a big wad of hundred dollar bills and flushing them. If you use injections that plump and paralyze you are experiencing the equivalent of doing just that.

Think that $2,000 or more for a tissue-tightening, frightfully painful Thermage treatment is any different? In addition to flushing the money down the drain, you are putting yourself through needless torture for the remote possibility that you will hopefully look younger once the promised effects actually occur.

What are you hoping to gain?

If you wish for a younger looking face, you will have to change your thinking because having your face injected, cut, sutured or deeply heated with an electrical device will not return your face to the look you remember.

The face you desire is your face ten to fifteen years ago.

When your fresh face began to fail you, you probably ran first to the drugstore, then to the dermatologist and you found your way to plastic surgery just hoping that the lotions, potions and their bag of tricks could somehow return the face you remembered.

You know the one: tight forehead, no wrinkles vertically or horizontally, bright open eyes with no visible crow's feet, nasal labial folds and marionette lines were not a possibility and that dreaded wattle was only worn by dear Aunt Joan. Your face was so beautiful and you loved everything about you.

Now the look of old is quickly appearing and you realize that even after willingly spending thousands and thousands of dollars on vanity serums with several nips and tucks, liposuction and more, you could easily spend that amount again and never see the end in sight.

How depressing!

Perhaps this is a blessing in disguise. Consider this: just how many injections of paralyzing and plumping chemicals can your face endure before it begins to look a little freakish? How many cuts and sutures can your face tolerate before you are wearing the wind-tunnel look? And, the other modalities offered may contribute to speeding up the aging process when indeed they promise to help you look younger.

What if these menus of services are just a bunch of hooey designed to lighten your wallet time and time again because the aging process continues no matter which method you choose.

Sagging facial features are not very attractive and if you have doubts that using expensive "quick fix solutions" may not produce the desired results while you frivolously spend your hard earned cash your thinking is on track.

There is a safe and sane solution that deals directly with droopy facial features. A simple facial exercise program will tighten, contour and lift your face.

Isometric and resistance training works for the body and the same principles will work for the face.

Fingers, thumbs and white cotton gloves are all you need to lift sagging eyebrows, cheeks, jowls, pouches and more. These movements that require only 35 seconds each can be performed in the privacy of your home; you don't need to purchase any special equipment nor do you have to make an appointment with a licensed professional to enjoy spectacular results that can have you looking ten to fifteen years younger in less time than you thought possible.

For long-term beauty it is evident that facial exercise is superior to cuts, sutures and injections. Faces that forego these costly invasive procedures and opt instead for natural beauty through exercise will never look hard, done or over done.

One final point: we have all seen photos of plastic surgery gone wrong. It could happen to you even if you have carefully chosen the ideal practitioner. When you see celebrities' face work that isn't quite right, please remind yourself that they can afford the very best but their results do not always portray a younger look. What can you expect?

With facial exercise there are no surprises, you look like you only better!

Facial Exercise or Botox

Once the Hippocratic Oath was considered a rite of passage for practitioners of medicine; it was a promise traditionally taken by physicians pertaining to the ethical practice of medicine. Over the years the wording has changed to reflect a more modern language; however, an oath of some type is uttered by most physicians accepting the responsibility to practice medicine or is it to practice responsible medicine?

Botox, Restylane and Collagen are the darlings of many cosmetic surgeons' because these products create a huge cash flow upsurge that boosts their bottom line. These same products provide a very temporary result that requires multiple treatments every year; most patients, mainly women, are willing to continue the injections giving no thought to how their faces will look or behave if they stop using these crutches.

A FDA article says, "In 2001, more than 1.6 million people received injections, an increase of 46 percent over the previous year. More popular than breast enhancement surgery and a potential blockbuster, Botox is regarded by some as the ultimate fountain of youth." On the other hand, the FDA describes Botox Cosmetic as a toxin. HTTP://www.fda.gov/bbs/topics/ANSWERS/2002/ANS01147.html Updating the figure for injections, Botox led the way in 2005.

Should there be concern for over-treatment or abuse when it comes to using these products? The above referenced FDA article echoes concern that Botox use could be easily abused, especially when untrained and unqualified people are doing the injecting at $500 a treatment. Abuse also comes when the patient complains to the care giver that the treatment was not as effective as promised so the injection is repeated before the recommended waiting period has lapsed.

If the results of a typical injection last 120 days, that means a patient returns at least three times per year to repeat the procedure to maintain that paralyzed look. At what point does a patient reach saturation with these drugs? One-tenth of a teaspoon, the typical amount of product used for the forehead, doesn't sound like much in terms of product usage but the burning question remains: what is the long-term ramification of injecting a toxin into the body several times a year?

Most cosmetic Botox injections target the forehead lines, the concentration lines between the brows and the area around the eyes. These particular lines and creases indicate that the underlying muscles have lost elasticity and tone from atrophy coupled with continued repetitive motion. Yes, the motion needs to be stopped but surprisingly, stopping the learned behavior of frowning or raising the forehead when emoting requires behavior modification not paralyzing toxins.

There is a non-invasive, all natural remedy for muscles that are lax – it's not an injection and it's not a cream. It's exercise! Exercise using isometric and resistance movements can easily tighten the underlying muscles of the face and neck. Imagine, learning a series of exercise motions that you can use forever and the results can stave off the need for injections because the underlying muscles will plump up and become strong again. When the muscles are made stronger, the skin feels and acts like younger skin.

Botox is not the Fountain of Youth – it is a toxin that blocks the release of a chemical by nerve cells that signal muscle contraction. When normal muscle contraction is inhibited, new wrinkles can begin their formation. That's right - New wrinkles are developed when compensating for other muscles lack of movement.

Exercise for the face can keep the underlying muscles strong so that wrinkles are less likely to form. Why resort to man-made chemicals when exercise can help you look younger and healthier?

Remember, beauty injections do not cure; they only temporarily mask the symptoms.

Love Your Face – Don't Inject It Or Mutilate It!

Looked in the mirror lately only to see a misshapen face that has hooded eyes, sagging cheeks and a double chin looking back at you? Maybe even today you lifted the skin up and back and wished it would stay that way.

If this is the sad state of your face, you may unwisely believe that only injections or plastic surgery can save it. You would be wrong!

Facial exercise has long been touted as the safest, most reliable remedy for sagging facial features because it is natural and cannot do harm. Just like exercise works for your arms, legs, torso and body, facial exercise can indeed create a newer looking face in just minutes a day.

That's right, in just minutes a day you can control the look of aging in your face using specialized facial exercises designed to tighten, lift and firm up sagging muscles and skin.

Droopy cheeks, down turned mouth corners, even that dreaded wattle can be chiseled when you learn how to create strong facial muscles. Muscles that weave over and under each other lose their elasticity by the time your face is 40 and by age 55, you can believe those muscles have elongated at least one-half inch.

Elongated muscles show up on our arms as jiggly arms. Inner thigh muscles soften due to muscle atrophy. We either begin wearing clothing that covers up our out of shape bodies or we hit the gym and begin a fitness routine.

It seems that most of society has begun to sit up and take notice that diet and exercise are vitally important to our vitality. People are out moving around; they walk, jog, lift weights, and go to Yoga classes, Pilate's classes, spinning classes, and more to keep their body in better shape so that it purrs and runs smoothly for years and years.

The face has been forgotten. Oh sure, there are plenty of skin care items that would like for you to believe their hype – an eye lift from a jar, fillers for wrinkles and diffusers that illuminate the skin. Skin care will not lift sagging muscles. There is no such thing as a face lift from a jar. Neither can you stand on your head nor lie on your back long enough so that your facial muscles do not sag.

Your personal appeal is centered around your face. When people see you, they look at your face then make assumptions regarding your health and well being just by looking at your eyes, your mouth corners and your expressions.

If you indulge in risky behavior when it comes to your face, you may end up disgruntled, disfigured or even dead.

Risky surgeries and procedures occur daily. This is because some-one elects to do something drastic to change or alter their appearance without fully weighing all the consequences of using surgery or injec-tions to look younger.

These pathways of surgery and using injections that plump and para-lyze the face have not been fully explored by the scientists who develop the procedures and the serums. Scary but true. Most injections used by the medical community have not had extensive testing to show results for long-term use. Long term use is considered six months or more; if you are considering using Botox for your frown lines and you use the serum for over six months, you are pretty much on your own insofar as long use complications.

These quick fixes are not reliable methods but only temporary mea-sures that act as a stop gap; they do nothing to stop aging in the face.

Using exercise stops aging and as long as you continue to exercise your face a few minutes a day several times per week, you could look ten to fifteen years younger than your peers for a very long time.

There's no expensive equipment to buy to perform these highly spe-cialized movements. All you need are your thumbs and fingers and your white cotton gloves. And, don't forget your camera – be certain you take photos before you begin so you can see how far you have come in just nine weeks. You'll soon forget that you once had sagging cheeks, hooded eyes and a turkey wattle that made you look and feel older.

Sticking a Needle in Your Face is Invasive

Looking younger is the mantra of Baby Boomers. This generation and the subsequent generations have greatly contributed to the gold-filled pockets of plastic surgeons everywhere. The Botox and Restylane craze has never been more evident than in today's society. Aging just isn't what it used to be; now there is a plethora of anti-aging products for every price range that make lots of promises. What happened to aging gracefully?

Over and over again, the phrase "non-invasive" is touted but having injections, whether they're in your arm, your buttocks or your face is invasive. An injection requires a needle and when it is shoved into your skin, it is an invasion.

Yes, having an injection rather than a full-blown surgical procedure is non-surgical. There are many, many doctors and other practitioners who want consumers to believe that little doses of cadaver material or botulism injected in the forehead, the outer eye area and around the mouth, is not invasive but let's tell it like it is.

On a recent network morning show, two women, moms in their 40's, were willing to undergo "non-invasive procedures" to look younger. While the noted dermatologist took her black marker and began drawing on the faces to demonstrate how Botox and other material would be injected into certain areas to fill out and alleviate visible signs of aging, it was striking to see just how desperate these housewives have become. These injections would have cost at least $1500 - $2000 for a procedure that will have to be repeated at least twice during a one-year period of time if they want to maintain their results.

The quest for slowing down the aging process has become a multi-billion dollar business and in 2004, over 9 million cosmetic procedures were performed. Even though the effects of injections are gone in a short amount of time and plastic surgery requires updating, patients, particularly women, may have fallen into a trap believing that these procedures are the only avenue of preserving their looks.

There are other ways to turn back the clock without surgery or invasive injections and one is exercise, facial exercise. Exercising your face will restore the tone and firmness that you thought may have been lost forever. There is no recovery time, no risks of any type and you won't end up with the face of a stranger.

Crow's feet are a major concern because eyes look tired when these pesky little lines are apparent. The reason they form is because the forehead muscle has elongated due to gravity and life; when this happens, the muscles surrounding the eyes become compressed by the gravitational weight on them.

There is an easy remedy to alleviate the look of crow's feet: Place the three middle fingers of each hand underneath each eye brow. Push the eyebrows up and slightly outward. Hold your eyebrows high and begin to use your forehead muscle to push down into your fingertips. (Make certain you are not creating lines between your eyebrows; push outward towards the temple area after pushing up) Count slowly to five. Remove your hands, take a deep breath, and again position your fingertips underneath your brows. Push the eyebrows up and slightly outward. Hold them high and begin to use your forehead muscle to push down into your fingertips. Count to ten – at count 7, close your eyes. (This action forces oxygenated blood to the eye lids) Remove your hands and repeat this two more times for a total of thirty-five seconds of exercise. If this exercise is performed once a day for six days in a row, in less than three weeks, the eyebrows will have lifted and crow's feet will be less noticeable.

See how easy that was and you saved $3500! You can lift your entire face and neck with simple isometric/resistance exercises that require thirty five seconds for each movement. No pain, no anesthesia, no risk and great results – at home and in hardly any time at all.

Will Bangs Replace Botox?

Ever wonder how your face will look in ten years? If so, there's a scary way to determine just how well those hidden muscles beneath the skin are holding up: Place a mirror flat on your vanity, bend over from the waist and as you peer at your face, slowly count to ten. See, I told you it could be scary.

Aging in the face is very subtle; the gradual loosening of muscles, the lack of collagen production, the formation of wrinkles and hollows will all become apparent as Mother Nature continues her march across our faces. Maybe you've noticed the vertical lines deepening, the horizontal lines firmly etching outwards to the temples and now crow's feet are firmly in place. This type of aging is all about lax muscles.

Just as you have seen changes in your upper arms, waist, tummy, hips and thighs, these same changes occur throughout the body and this includes the face. A lack of exercise can make our body look and feel older than our years.

We can cleverly camouflage certain body flaws but disguising an aging face is another matter.

What looks like aging to you? Is it environmental circumstances such as over exposure to the sun, wind and smog? Is it pursed lips? Does your skin look old because you didn't wash your face every night and now hormonal changes present their own dry skin challenges with fine lines turning into wrinkles? Maybe your face has become spongy and droopy; has it elongated and headed south?

Wearing sagging facial muscles is wearing the look of old.

Yes, this is aging at its worst and it is happening to everyone. For those of you over the age of 25, this is a stark reality. No matter what your age, you have choices to make regarding your good health and how you age gracefully.

Lots of professionals have jumped on the anti-aging bandwagon. Drug and pharmaceutical companies now provide physicians' lots of ammunition in the form of injections and skin care items using toxins, waxes, dyes, synthetics, etc.

The glossy magazines overflow with ads touting the latest and greatest skin care remedies that promise to tighten, lift and tone sagging skin. Maybe you have tried some of these products just hoping that one will actually change your facial appearance.

The choices are vast and varied. Some treatments and options are passive, others are aggressive and some are downright painful, risky and expensive.

If you love your body you have most likely decided that extreme measures are not for you. Maybe you have decided that wearing bangs is the best option. After all long bangs can disguise the lines and wrinkles or can they?

Botox came on the scene a few years ago with their very popular Botulinum A-Toxin injections that indeed paralyze and weaken injected muscles. The crippling of the muscles does result in smoothed foreheads and deters the look of crow's feet because the muscle movements are inhibited.

Even though relatively small amounts of this toxin are used, the body may or may not exhibit side effects but there are always side effects associated with every drug. There are those unlucky ones who do suffer certain physical consequences when allowing this toxin to be injected for cosmetic purposes such as overdose, misinjection, weakness, paralysis, and more.

The FDA has approved Botox for certain uses but due to recent information regarding the safety aspect of this drug, a black box warning may be issued which means that if you decide to allow this toxin to be injected, you will be duly warned by the administering physician. Scary indeed!

If you decline to use paralyzing toxins what options other than bangs do you have to either disguise or stop the lines and wrinkles in the forehead?

What if you were given isometric exercises to thwart the ravages of forehead lines and wrinkles? Would you be interested in knowing there is a proven, natural way to correct facial sagging so that your face returns to a more youthful, contoured appearance?

When the forehead develops lines and wrinkles, it is because the broad, vertical frontalis muscle is losing its intrinsic tone; this muscle elongates and pushes downward into the eyebrow muscles and upper eye. This action creates compression as muscles pool into each other.

The entire face and the neck can become misshapen when the facial muscles no longer provide adequate support of the skin. Just like your body appreciates exercise to maintain its sleekness and form, the facial muscles also benefit from isometric movements.

This action of the exercise forces oxygenated blood to the tissues; from the inside out your face and neck will look more vibrant and alive in hardly any time at all while your muscles plump up and support your skin without harmful interventions.

Bangs? Well, only if they're in style but you'll no longer need to wear them to disguise your forehead when you use exercise to keep your face looking younger. Imagine surgery-like results without a knife, injection, inconvenience, expense or pain.

Young Women Who Use Cosmetic Procedures Fare Better With Facial Exercise

Many young women, those under the age of 30, flock to the cosmetic counters in droves so they can experiment with colors for every season, moods for evening and natural and not so natural looks for daytime. The kaleidoscope is very enticing as department store after department store, drug store after drug store, boutiques and cosmetic super-stores vie for sales of every type and kind of topical enhancements.

Fueled by slick, artful, colorful advertising in magazines and billboards, it is easy to understand how enticing the allure of beauty has permeated our lives.

There is certainly nothing wrong with wanting to look as pretty as possible; after all, your face is your calling card, your power suit and for a very long time, it is a well-known fact that a beautiful face is a powerful asset - an asset that can propel a woman through the glass ceiling and beyond when her brains and IQ transcend the stratosphere.

Sometimes the lines blur and the once easy-breezy attitude regarding aging begins to shift.

All of sudden, it seems, a trip to the cosmetic counter just isn't enough. No matter which foundation, blush, eye shadow or mascara is used, visible signs of aging have appeared and nothing seems to work.

All you want is to restore your once fabulous face and stop the droopy eyes, jowls and slightly sagging skin.

Perhaps drastic interventions such as injections of Botox, Restylane, Perlane, Juviderm, and Collagen have been considered. Even the thought of plastic surgery may seem attractive as worry and fear over the future of a once young looking face is indeed very real.

It is unfortunate that these invasive and risky procedures are considered viable to correct the visible signs of aging. Plumping and paralyzing, cutting and suturing do not stop or correct sagging facial muscles. Interventions of injections and surgery only temporarily mask aging.

When a young woman chooses these modalities first, she has forever changed the natural, youthful face she craves because injections, full of toxins and chemicals, are unnatural to the body and no one really knows or understands the long-term ramifications of using these untested drugs. The body does not readily integrate these foreign substances and your system begins to work very hard to rid the body of these toxins.

Once a person becomes a slave to nips and tucks or injections that plump and paralyze the facial features, it is unlikely that the face will ever look youthful; rather it is common that the face just looks "unnaturally done".

Young women, heed this advice: if you want to maintain a youthful face stay out of the plastic surgeon's office because once you go through that door, their job is to provide you with an alluring anti-aging menu to keep you as a patient for a very long time.

At first you may just acquiesce to deep cleaning and facials but it won't be long until you have 'graduated' to more extensive procedures - like plumping and paralyzing - while laying out lots of cash for temporary fixes that may not produce the desired results.

What are your desired results? Don't you just want to look like you did ten to fifteen years ago? Well, you can when you use facial exercise, a safe, no risk method that strengthens the facial muscles and rejuvenates the face.

Facial muscles support the facial skin. If you see loosening and sagging, it is because the muscles are softening and soon they will begin to pool into other muscles. This is when wrinkles will begin to form.

You may or may not know that facial muscles can elongate up to one half inch by the time your face is 55. We see the changes in our arms, waist, tummy, hips and thighs that began in our early 30's. We learn to mask the flaws with clothing.

The best anti-aging defense for a face that is showing signs of fatigue via sagging facial muscles is the very pro-active, proven method of facial exercise that will lift tone and tighten droopy facial features.

Exercise works for the body and exercise can sculpt and contour your facial features.

Facial exercise is deep muscle conditioning that does not use contortions, twists, puckers and scrunches. If you scrunch or twist or contort your face hoping to see lifting and toning, you will be disappointed. This type of exercise may even increase and accentuate existing lines and wrinkles.

The type of exercise most beneficial for the face is isometric with resistance movements. This means you learn to position your thumbs and fingers to simply anchor the muscle. The next movement you learn contracts the muscle. The muscles respond by repositioning.

These easy movements that require only minutes a day to complete are valuable because once you learn the techniques, they are yours for life. Your face can look substantially younger in hardly any time at all when you use these face saving techniques.

For those of you who are searching the cosmetic counters, considering a risky procedure or even a nip, tuck, looking refreshed, radiant and natural is the most wonderful by-product of using facial exercise. You have the best advantage over aging with long lasting results and all without harm.

Career

Can Facial Exercise Boost Your Career?

Safe, sane exercise wins again as nips and tucks have been outed. Speeding up the aging process is just another contraindication of surgery. That's right, if you choose surgery, and allow your beautiful healthy face to be cut; your face may never look youthful again due to skin discoloration, unnatural draping and evident scarring.

Self improvement schemes that involve cutting, suturing and injecting may put your face on a fast track to look older.

Here's why: once you begin injecting with paralyzing and plumping serums or using surgery that cuts and discards bits and pieces of your skin, muscle and more, it is likely that you may not realize that your face is still aging.

That is because the aging process continues no matter how many surgeries are performed and no matter how many injections are used.

Ladies and gentlemen, save your money, your time and your sanity if you want to look somewhat normal when you approach your golden years because years of abuse and self mutilation will take its toll no matter if it's surgery, liposuction or injections.

The media has artfully crafted stories that most likely are carefully spun tales from the surgery proponents that woo you into believing that if you do not partake of their wares, something is wrong. Their message is that your job, your very existence relies on your surgically altered, paralyzed and plumped, laser surfaced face.

Surgery and injections just don't cut it anymore and they should be the very last resort when you are contemplating creating a younger looking face. Weighing all the options just got easier!

Of course looking your best is in the competitive business market is a great asset and it's good to remember that you bring more to the table than just a pretty face; however, when you realize that your face could look healthier, less stressed, less droopy, you could benefit from learning a simple exercise routine that acts to turn back the clock with noticeable results.

Facial exercise works best to tackle sagging facial muscles. Rather than cutting tissue, exercise plumps up the facial muscles. Exercised facial muscles support your skin because exercise nourishes your skin with oxygenated blood. This returns the look of young to your face.

Results from exercise are more reliable than surgery and injections. You will look like yourself only a younger version and there will be no scars, no risk and no surprises. People will still recognize you and your results will amaze even your closest friends.

Exercise requires only a few minutes each time you work-out your face. You really do not need any special equipment although special exercise gloves will definitely aid in anchoring and positioning your thumbs and fingers so that when you grasp a muscle there is no chance of slipping.

Slow, deliberate exercise motions will lift, sculpt and tighten your facial features.

Muscles that are exercised exhibit new life; you see sleekness develop in your waist, tummy, hips and thighs. You see sculpting and contouring occur and this gives your body a new look. The very same principles apply for the face when you use contraction and resistance exercise to reclaim your face.

Gravity plays a big part in how your face looks today. So does loss of fat.

By exercising the facial muscles, you will notice how your smile is enhanced when the cheek muscles reposition to a much younger stance. Your eyes will appear more open as your frontalis muscle, the forehead muscle, begins to shorten and tighten. Exercise can tighten, sculpt and lift your neck, the wattle, jowls, pouches, lower and upper cheeks, crows feet, horizontal and vertical lines on the forehead and between the eye brows.

Your entire face will feel the newness that is developed each time you perform the exercises and the excitement is real because you know you can recapture that younger face you thought was lost forever.

Easy, simple exercises that you complete in just minutes a day can transform your face into a younger looking you. Your confidence level will soar when you realize you save thousands of dollars, preserve your good looks and look 10-15 years younger.

Face Lift and Eye Lid Surgery: A Career Investment

Recently an article crossed my desk describing how a 45-50 year old male attorney began hearing remarks from his colleagues that he looked tired. Even though his suit was meticulous, starched collar and silk tie – he felt great but his facial appearance had begun to wane.

Consider this: A tall, shapely woman confidently dressed in form-fitting leotards and tights working out in her favorite spa. From the back view she looks like a 20 something – nothing jiggles – her waist, tummy, and thighs all in proportion. But as she turns, you see the tired, stressed out face of a definitely 40ish or older woman desperately trying to hold on to her youth.

This scenario represents the graying of the Baby Boomers; they see aging faces developing right before their eyes and they feel helpless thinking that they, too, may have to succumb to a surgical procedure to maintain the look of health and youthfulness as a career investment.

Will they need a mini-lift? Eye lid surgery? Liposuction on their chin and neck? Not so long ago, "nips and tucks" were quiet affairs and only available to celebrities and business moguls' wives; today plastic surgery is becoming mainstream as more and more financing options become available. Business execs, sales people, secretaries, practically every one over the age of 20 realize that their facial appearance speaks volumes about themselves: Furrowed brows: angry and explosive. Down Turned Mouth Corners: looks sad, maybe depressed Double Chin & Jowls: Looks old - old ideas.

Surgical procedures are risky. There is not one procedure performed under the guise of plastic surgery that is risk-free. Not only does a patient risk infection from an invasive procedure; scarring and loss of sensation are also a concern. There have been cases where people have suffered brain damage from anesthesia and some have died.

At what point is seeking improvement detrimental? With so many procedures available, one has to ask if the medical community has slipped into an "assembly line" status.

These very serious surgeries may disfigure one's face and body as witnessed in many recent television shows portraying botched procedures. Noses, breasts, chins implants, liposuction nightmares and faces that look distorted cost someone a lot of cash and emotional anguish.

Imagine, paying hard earned money for a look that you may not embrace and maybe paying more to correct something that may need to be tweaked. Once tissue has been cut and sutured, it is never the same. Susan Sarandon, in a rare moment of candor, expressed succinctly to Ellen DeGeneres, "I'm scared of plastic surgery. You're somewhere between a burn victim and a female impersonator, and then there's a kind of an Asian thing going on."

What if the procedure goes smoothly; there are no problems and the patient is satisfied with the new look? How long will this investment last? Most facial plastic surgery procedures, especially injections, will have to be repeated again and again. Imagine facing another surgery —

anesthesia and more cutting can eventually disfigure a face. The average surgical procedure is $20,000. Multiple expenditures can quickly add up to staggering amounts.

More and more people are opting for non-surgical methods of facial rejuvenation; in fact, just as isometric and resistance type exercise works to reshape the body, facial exercise can significantly reverse the look of aging in every face. Here's how: As we age, muscles in the face slowly relax and as they relax your skin begins to follow the downward motion. Jowls and little pouches form on the jaw line, the eyelids begin to fold and a visible line develops in your cheeks between your nose and mouth.

Unlike the major muscles in the body, the facial muscles are small; in some areas they weave over and under each other, and they attach at only one end to a bone. This means they cannot contract without an artificial anchor – in our arms and legs, we have joints that act as anchors so that we can tense our muscles with contractions. In order to contract the facial muscles so they tone, tighten and lift they must be held or anchored. This action provides increased circulation and oxygenation. This means that contortions – movements without resistance – will not contour the face and neck. Resistance exercise lifts your face from the inside out.

Using resistance and isometric movements will reshape and lift your face. These exercises create stronger, more resilient muscles and facial skin will tighten preventing further sagging. The jowls will lift, eyes will open and look vibrant and the "apples" in your cheeks will return. With exercise, you can look younger and people will recognize you even if you haven't seen them in twenty years because you will still look like you.

Recession-Proof Your Face

If your face has stopped you from looking in the mirror because you cannot fathom how in the world your face could droop and sag in so many directions; just know that you are not alone.

After all aging happens and if you don't see apparent signs that your facial features, your arms and hips are sliding south by age 35, you are very fortunate that your parents and grandparents gifted you with youthful genes.

For those of us who have discovered droopy eyelids, sagging cheeks and the dreaded wattle, there is hope that easily surpasses the "mainstream, quick-fix, big bucks solutions for a youthful face."

Temporary, paralyzing and plumping, toxin-laden injections produce a weird, freakish, unnatural contour to faces; they cost a lot of money and do nothing to promote good health or make a face look younger.

The truth is hard to hear: using made-made substances that claim to prop up sagging skin will not last. Oh sure, you will initially see a difference but the reality is this: injections, like surgeries, must be consistently repeated and refreshed ala Joan Rivers. Now Joanie has pretty deep pockets and can easily afford to keep her plastic surgeon driving a Maserati in Marbella; but, can you?

Economic considerations aside - relying on frivolous, risky modalities means you give away your power; where is your commitment to a healthy mind, body and soul? Tied to the end of a syringe or a scalpel?

Are you willing to become the gerbil on the wheel, a slave to temporary measures that may corrupt your long-term good health and deplete your savings?

How many injections, surgeries, lipo-suctions and treatments can your body handle without rebelling? New reports suggest that aggressive and invasive anti-aging procedures actually speed-up aging so be advised that prolonged use of injections and more may not produce the desired effects.

Consider celebrities who readily invest money in the best of everything - homes, vacations, travel, and luxury de jour - have by choice chosen plastic surgery, injections and loads of treatment just hoping to further enhance their appearance, career, and bankability. Without naming names, we have seen results that surely weren't anticipated.

Oversized lips, ghastly raised eyebrows, inflated cheeks, splayed mouths, flat cheeks, the wind-tunnel, surprised look coupled with harsh laser treatments that guarantee any face could easily resemble the Bride of Frankenstein are frequently seen in the hottest spots like the Ivy and Nobu, in gossip magazines and celebrity blogs. If celebrities who can afford the finest of everything end up with freakish looking faces, what will you get?

You can easily recession-proof your face and look younger than your years if you are willing to try an all-natural alternative like facial exercise.

Exercise changes everything. Just as torsos, arms, legs, hips, buttocks and thighs slim and tighten with regular exercise; facial exercise can tighten and lift the sagging facial features that make a face look tired and old.

Rather than spending several thousand dollars on temporary fixes invest in a facial exercise program to manage your sagging cheeks and eyebrows, double chins, lined foreheads and more.

Don't be fooled thinking all facial exercise programs are the same. Facial exercise that employs resistance and isometric movements go far beyond contortions, twitches and scrunches to insure that your face will lift, tighten and contour.

Once you learn the simple movements, you are highly unlikely to darken the doctor's door holding a syringe filled with chemicals because your forehead will tighten, your eyes will lift, your cheeks will not sag and you will look like yourself again only years younger.

Facial exercise requires only minutes a day to complete a routine. Your thumbs and fingers clothed in white cotton gloves accurately target those small sagging underlying muscles. Those muscles will feel alive again in just seconds as oxygenated blood that distributes nutrients to our cells courses through the tissues.

Not only will facial exercise restore the muscle tone in your face and neck, your confidence will soar. You can dance all the way to the bank because your clever new beauty regime didn't cost you a bundle and you feel alive and well knowing that no foreign or toxic substance was injected into your body.

Imagine, a younger looking face without the danger, risk or unpredictability of injections, drugs or surgery using all natural exercise.

Cheeks

Sagging Cheeks -
Lift Using Facial Exercises

How many times did you stand in front of your mirror this week only to gently lift the sides of your face up and back into the hairline? This futile action may have temporarily "lifted" your appearance but if you want to have lasting results, those sagging cheek muscles need a rescue regime and they need it now.

Full, beautiful cheeks are vital to a youthful face. Nasal labial folds develop when the mid face begins to sag; facial muscles droop and pool into other muscles and muscle groups creating the look of old.

Sagging cheeks portray a clear indication that the muscles in the face no longer adequately support the skin; that downward slide elongates your face in subtle ways. At first you may notice fine lines developing and a slight shift in your facial appearance may be evident only to you; but you know what is happening, don't you? This is aging and it won't stop ever.

The upper and lower face muscles weave over and under each other; one end attaches to bone in the skull and the other muscle end attaches either to another muscle or directly into the skin. As these muscles soften from disuse, the fullness of your face is affected as jowls, pouches and sagging cheeks develop.

Atrophied, softened muscles drag down your skin to form the look of old we dread. It isn't so funny when you see Great Aunt Hilda's chin developing below your jaw. Hereditary or not, sagging cheeks, double chins and more quickly add up to wearing a matronly face.

Men and women worldwide share the desire to maintain a youthful face. In our youth-obsessed society, wrong or right, a beautiful or handsome face often seems to enjoy special attention and more interest but youthfulness can wane.

There was a time that anti-aging options were limited to mostly skin care lotions and potions, facials, lasers, injections and surgery.

Now that consumers are savvy to the fact that these temporary modalities require repeated maintenance updates and refreshment, more and more patients realize that their hard earned money is not well spent. After all, who wants to frequently inject costly, synthetic chemicals and fillers that carry dire warnings and partake in dangerous surgical alterations when it is well-known that these measures attribute to aging?

In addition to wrecking your skin there is evidence that many adverse reactions occur in the weeks and months following invasive procedures such as injections and surgeries. These potential complications can include allergic reactions, swelling, inflammatory reactions that result in nodule formation, cold sores, arthritis and other immune challenges, infection, bruising, bleeding, blisters, cysts, lumps, bumps, numbness and migration issues.

Remember, you may not see complications immediately but they can rear their ugly head at any time after the initial procedure has been completed.

Buying risky injections and submitting to dicey surgeries can challenge your senses when you realize that you no longer recognize the face reflected in your mirror.

Even in the best case scenarios, when everything goes perfectly, eventually you will be faced with 'revision decisions' because it won't be long until you recognize the subtle shifting and you are faced with more injections and surgery.

Do you feel like a gerbil yet?

What if plastic surgery and injections were obsolete?

How surprised would you be to learn that sagging cheeks, droopy necks, jowls and pouches do not require surgical intervention or fillers that plump and injections that paralyze?

There is a way to tighten your face and lift your features using specialized contouring and isometric contractions that require only a few minutes of your time with results that rival the face you loved ten to fifteen years ago.

Here's how this happens: Thumbs and fingers in white cotton exercise gloves are easily manipulated into movements, think resistance and contraction, that work to sculpt your facial muscles.

A droopy face indicates that muscles are shifting and pooling into other muscles and muscle groups; when certain specific isometric exercise contractions are used, muscles "awaken" and begin to return to their more youthful shape. The skin is revitalized as beneficial nutrients via oxygenated blood are unleashed, the muscles plump up and the face looks younger.

Repositioning the underlying muscles means you can wear a younger looking face. Manipulating lax facial muscles, then seeing and feeling them respond, will dramatically enhance your good looks and elevate your confidence level.

Slow yet deliberate exercise movements are taught first for the heaviest muscles in the face and neck. Week One teaches you how to successfully contract the upper cheek and the upper eye muscles. These two actions will noticeably improve the smoothness of your skin while lifting the cheeks, forehead and upper eyes. These two exercises require thirty-five seconds each.

You don't have to go anywhere or buy special equipment - these treatments are done in the privacy of your home.

Week Two begins by performing the two exercises learned in Week One and then adding two new actions that address the lower cheeks and lower mouth - firming and lifting the jowls and pouches. Performing these four exercises requires only seconds of your time. From the beginning your face will feel more toned and lifted and soon your reflection in the mirror will reveal changes.

Over the next seven weeks you will teach yourself the simple yet easy steps to keep your face looking toned and younger. Neck, double chin, the dreaded wattle, under eyes, upper lips, crow's feet and more can be enhanced when you realize that the power of looking younger is in your hands.

Mindful, proactive, safe, sane and natural methods will assure that you age spectacularly. Smiling never felt so good! And, your cheeks? Wowee Zowee!

Chin

Double Chins Remedied Using Facial Exercise

When you closely examine your face what is the biggest detraction or the neon light that calls attention to your facial imperfections? Is that looming chin - the dreaded wattle - tops on your list?

Double chins can occur even when you haven't gained an ounce but wearing an extra roll of flesh can make you look pounds heavier.

Covering your body when your waist, tummy, arms or hips are expanding is a type of camouflage most girls learn at an early age. We can wear slimming clothes that detract from the actual challenges of gaining a few pounds; now with spandex undergarments, we can easily hide and disguise bulging waistlines or less than thin thighs.

Just as you see aging in other areas of your face such as hooded eyes, sagging cheeks and folds along your mouth, these are all indications that the once tight muscles hidden beneath your skin are now losing their firmness which results in a look reminiscent of your elder relatives.

It is not that you do not love and cherish Great Aunt Hilda or Grandpa Joe, you just do not want to look like them now.

Facial flaws are a distraction. They can make us appear older than our years and this saps our confidence whether we are in the dating scene, updating our resume or interacting with others.

Wearing a double chin cannot be disguised with turtlenecks or scarves. A double chin cannot be concealed with makeup or other cosmetic preparations. Double chins are a result of muscle atrophy. That's right - muscle atrophy as in no activity.

If the wearer is not overweight what is the remedy?

Liposuction for a double chin is one choice but spending thousands of dollars for an iffy procedure fraught with risks, bruising, swelling, lumps and bumps and temporary benefits may not seem likely for the discerning person. In addition you would want to consider that numbness and nerve damage, puckering at the incision site and scar tissue are lingering aspects associated with this procedure.

Liposuction after all goes after the fat but what if you have very little fat but a lot of sagging or bulging?

Sculpting a wayward chin with isometric exercise is a safe alternative and the results become noticeable quickly. Why? The underside of your chin and into the neck is comprised of a broad, flat muscle called the platysma. This large muscle acts like any other muscle that is not sufficiently exercised - it droops and sags as it slowly pools into other muscles and easily collects deposits of fat.

If the area under your chin feels soft, not toned or taut or you see an enlarged mass when you look at your profile, without a doubt, this is the start of a less than youthful look.

Sadly, over time, the entire face begins to soften and elongate.

You can prove this to yourself by placing a mirror flat on the table while bending over from the waist looking down into the mirror. Gaze at yourself for ten seconds to see just how dramatically soft your facial muscles are. I warn you, it is a scary look that alerts you that your facial features are losing their contour because the muscles that support the skin are no longer in great shape. This atrophy causes the look of old.

Fortunately, atrophy can be reversed and those tiny facial muscles can indeed grow stronger while your skin receives added nutrition from oxygenated blood that is created when you exercise your face.

Facial exercises that shorten, tighten, lift and contour your muscles are not contortions, twists or puckers; rather facial exercise that can help you look five, ten even fifteen years younger are a result of isometric with resistance type contractions.

Thumbs and fingers and cotton exercise gloves are all that is required for you to take charge of your aging face. Step-by-step you can begin to expertly manipulate your facial muscles so they respond easily to the movements and in just minutes a day you will feel and see the lifting and contouring.

Your sagging cheeks, droopy eye lids and double chin will show great improvement as the results last longer and longer. Your face will look and feel toned and tightened, your confidence will soar and before long you will challenge your friends to look in the mirror lying flat on the table.

Facial Exercise Melts Double Chins

Double chins are move prevalent now than ever before as people exhibit the telltale signs of weight gain. Yes, obesity is a world wide health epidemic and it affects more than just our waist lines.

Funny thing about our bodies...you can cover up a somewhat overweight body using loose clothes, black tops and slacks and even some long jackets can disguise body flaws but there is nothing that can camouflage that hanging flesh under our chins that absolutely ages every face.

Double chins are worn by both men and women, yet while wearing extra pounds of flesh may indeed be displayed under our jaw; sagging chins are the result of the extra weight impacting the very large, dense neck muscle.

If you see a double chin in your mirror, just know that your facial muscles are definitely sagging and elongating, too.

Facial muscles can elongate up to one-half inch by the time your face is 55 years old. This elongation gives you hooded eyes, sagging cheeks, jowls, pouches and the dreaded wattle can, over time, become a full-blown double chin.

Medical professionals would like you to believe that liposuction is the ideal solution to remedy a big chin that detracts from your good looks.

What if you cannot afford a large cash outlay? Maybe you have diabetes or take high blood pressure medication; did you know that certain medication might interfere with a successful procedure? Maybe you just cringe at the thought of someone manipulating a cannula under your skin. What about significant risk to your good health?

What if you choose liposuction and you do not like the results? What can you do about dents and lumps? What if your results look unnatural? What is your remedy? Do you hope the surgeon will refund your money? That is highly unlikely.

Many people who desire a younger looking face have decided to choose a path that involves an all natural, alternative method - one that does not create health risks and one that guarantees that you will look exactly like yourself only younger and certainly recognizable.

This alternative method is facial exercise that uses resistance and isometric contraction of the muscles. When these methods are employed, the facial muscles strengthen and lift, creating a more youthful face in just hardly any time at all.

Most medical practitioners have been leery to recommend facial exercise to their clients because many programs consist of twists, puckers, contortions and movements of the face that are mostly laughable. Everyone would indeed be right to avoid those unlikely expressions because repetitive movements can accentuate existing lines and wrinkles. Repeated contortions might even create lines and wrinkles.

Using isometric with resistance facial exercise applies the same principles to the face that are used for the body. This type of exercise training plumps up the muscles and muscle groups with oxygenated blood, the skin acts youthful and a new smoothness develops in your face.

Will you look like you did at 20? Not exactly but you will enjoy an improved, lifted, and tightened face and neck. That double chin will begin to melt away as muscles strengthen and return to a more youthful position.

Most plastic surgery procedures hope to help you look ten years younger but often the recipient of surgery only looks like they have had work done, not necessarily any younger. Surgery is risky business and economically there is a lot of money involved for temporary, risky procedures.

Facial exercise that uses resistance and isometric retraining of the facial muscles produces amazing results that can surpass facial plastic surgery results. Surgery creates flat, taut faces that usually look unnatural and if laser techniques are applied, faces appear shiny and eerie looking and possibly unrecognizable.

Injections that plump and paralyze facial features do not look natural; strings, electro-stimulation, and other modalities are not youthfully complimentary.

Your best bet to erase the years? Your thumbs and fingers. Anchoring facial muscles to generate a contraction is the ticket to a lifetime of facial fitness.

Imagine looking in the mirror after only a few weeks of using facial exercise to see a younger version of yourself peering back at you. That double chin and sagging face that caused a lack of self-confidence can be substantially eliminated using facial exercise for just minutes a day. Your self-esteem will soar and you will be delighted with your results.

Exercise is a very inexpensive modality that brings sustainable results. What do you have to lose? Only your tired, out of shape face. Just give it a try!

Eyes

A Quick Fix for Sagging, Heavy Eyelids

Droopy eyelids are a sure sign that Mother Nature has arrived to make your face look old.

You know the look and the feel of heavy lids - they seem to have a mind of their own. You constantly lift your forehead when you are speaking and your eyes may begin to feel a tiredness that just doesn't go away.

Not only are your eyes bothering you, those forehead wrinkles may have you thinking that a paralyzing injection might be required or even more drastic measures such as surgery may be needed.

The medical community wants you to believe that you need to consider this route to look younger but in reality – this is not a fact!

The upper eye lids, the brow and upper forehead are connected under the skin with muscles that weave over and under each other. The actual forehead muscle is vertical and it originates in the hairline.

Usually by age 40, gravity has affected the forehead resulting in poor muscle tone and its downward slide pushes into the eyebrow muscles which then affects the upper eye lid and creates crow's feet. This downward movement of loose skin can impair one's vision if the lid puddles onto the eyelashes.

There are only a few options available to enjoy younger looking eyes.

Blepharoplasty is a surgical procedure to correct sagging upper and lower eyes. The upper eye procedure involves actually cutting the eyelids, removing excess tissue and then suturing the eyelids usually in the existing crease. The surgery is performed while the patient is under general anesthesia although there are other types of local and oral anesthesias available; the procedure takes about 2 hours to complete and just like any other invasive procedure there are risks to consider.

Electro-stimulation devices, using minute electrical currents, claim they can lift eyelids and brows. According to some well-paid physicians they do work but there is a healthy amount of skepticism from their peers.

Overuse can cause spasms, headache, irritation, redness and burning. Electro-stimulation is very time consuming as each area requires about three minutes to treat so it's not unusual to spend an hour or more trying to lift your face every other day.

The above-mentioned options are not only costly; they're very temporary. Yes, temporary! Surgery does not correct poor muscle tone and neither do injections or electro-currents.

What's the solution?

Facial exercise is the smartest thing you can do to stop the cause of aging in your face but not all facial exercise programs work. Why? Because scrunching and contortions are not exercises!!! When there is no resistance or anchoring to create a contraction, your face cannot lift or look younger. Genuine facial exercise is not about scrunching or making contortions, rather, they are bone fide, precise movements that treat the cause of aging in your face.

How long until you see results? Well, most people see results immediately and you should know that it takes about three to four weeks to see permanent results. Permanent results occur when the muscles are sufficiently strengthened to retain their new positions. If you do not regularly exercise the muscles in the face, you will look older.

Our entire body needs exercise, and that includes our faces and necks. From head to toe, you can look healthier and vibrant without ever thinking about surgery, injections or electricity. Exercising your face requires only minutes per day and in less time than it took for your morning shower, you can have a face that looks 10-15 years younger.

Crow's Feet and How to Stop Them

Looking a little tired around your eyes lately and confused by the hype how to remedy those lines and wrinkles?

There are cosmetic companies touting products just hoping you will believe that crow's feet can be diminished just by rubbing a little pad around the eyes. And, some cosmetic companies would like you to spend a small fortune every month on a topical preparation filled with peptides and other substances to stop the smile movements that cause creasing.

Maybe you have considered more drastic measures like Botox or fillers to combat the look of old because you know that wrinkles shout to the world that you are not the fresh-faced beauty you once were.

Such silliness!

Crow's feet are caused when the forehead muscle, a large vertical muscle, begins to elongate and push downward into other muscle groups that surround the eyes. Couple this downward motion with smiling, squinting and other facial expressions and voila! You have lines and wrinkles in a very delicate area of the face.

Yes, while skin care is important, in most cases you will never need to go the route of surgery or injections that paralyze and plump to correct crow's feet. Treating crow's feet using extraneous methods such as laser and Thermage seems barbaric, potentially dangerous and useless because these methods do not stop the cause of Crow's feet; these modalities only temporarily mask the symptoms.

You can prove this to yourself when you choose facial exercise to look younger and prettier. In one movement you can increase the distance between your eye brows and eye lashes; you will also experience the amazement that when you perform this exercise your forehead lifts and tightens, too.

Exercise changes everything because it revitalizes your body and it can revitalize your facial features. Oxygenated blood can be forced to our tissues when we use isometric and resistance movements; this action plumps up the tissue and rejuvenates the muscles so they better support your skin.

Just so that you know, there are other facial exercises to combat an aging face so that your face is firmer and lifted without using anything but your age erasers - your thumbs and fingers - to create a younger looking, prettier face.

Rather than sitting in a physicians office for twenty minutes to two hours wasting time and spending money to have a treatment, you can self treat at home using just thirty-five seconds each day to stop your droopy forehead from creating unwanted lines, wrinkles and crinkles around your eyes. The benefits of facial exercise for this area are truly amazing because you will see and feel a substantial difference the first day you try the exercise.

Will you look like you're sixteen again? Probably not but if you want to stop the downward slide of your forehead without spending a fortune or putting yourself at risk, this is the ticket for which you have been searching.

It is important to note that once you begin exercising your upper eye and forehead muscles that you continue to do so once a day for six days in a row. Even though the time allowance seems slight, it is sufficient to lift that heavy, vertical muscle to alleviate the look of old.

Women even into their 80's have seen their crow's feet greatly diminish. Couple the forehead exercise with the one hundred circle exercise to reduce the lines and wrinkles caused by smiling and other facial expressions and you will begin to see that twinkle return to your eyes.

You may be scoffing at the thought of alleviating crow's feet without expensive interventions but I promise, you'll have the last laugh when you realize just how powerful facial exercise is to save your face.

Once the decompression of the forehead muscle is reversed, you can see that the area surrounding the eye acts differently. The area becomes lifted and tightened. Without anything invasive, pain, risk or expense, you can correct droopy facial features with simple, easy to perform movements that require only minutes a day to complete.

How long does it take to see results? Most everyone sees results the very first time the movements are performed; however, lasting results come at about three weeks into practicing this exercise. The more consistent you are, the better your results.

Capture your results on film or in a digital format; do this by taking close-up photos of your face before you begin. At the end of the third week, take another set of photos and see how the area has lifted and responded to this very special exercise.

Once you prove to prove to yourself that you don't need any special interventions to have a younger, prettier face, you might want to consider learning an isometric and resistance facial exercise program that will help you rediscover the face you thought you had lost forever.

What do you have to lose? Only the look of old!

How We Can Easily Correct Sagging Eyelids to Preserve Vision

Heavy eye lids may have looked sultry and sexy on long-gone film sirens like Bette Davis and Barbara Stanwyck but in today's society, heavy eye lids may mean that impaired vision is in your future.

Gravity plays a large role regarding the condition of your eye lids. Like the muscles in the body that elongate due inactivity and lack of exercise, your forehead and eye brows muscles can elongate, too, then move downward into the muscles surrounding the eyes.

This very quiet elongation means that one day you will notice that the distance between your eye brows and eye lashes have diminished and those once youthful eye lids look creased and lined.

Crows' feet are another indicator that your eye brows and forehead are in need of attention.

Crows' feet can be lines and they can also be folds that develop at the corner of the eye affecting the peripheral vision. Left untreated, you may consciously or unconsciously begin to lift your forehead when you are speaking resulting in deep horizontal forehead lines. You might also realize that you are experiencing eye strain, tiredness and even headaches from this increased activity.

Poor muscle tone and lack of ligament support that begins in the forehead will push downward into the brows and the results affect the eye lids as they pool onto the lashes resulting in impaired vision. This is caused by inactivity in the upper portion of the face.

Some people who have sagging eye lids, commonly called dermatochalasis by the medical community, will immediately elect to have surgery; some may even try Botox or other modalities recommended by their physician; however, there is another avenue that will produce remarkable results without anything invasive.

Rather than electing to have a brow lift or upper eye lid surgery or both, many savvy consumers are rethinking surgery and considering specialized facial exercise to correct this malady that usually affects most everyone over the age 50.

Just as exercise trims a thick waistline, slims inner and outer thighs and strengthens the abs, specific exercises can indeed lift sagging upper eyes, eye brows and more.

The forehead muscle is called the frontalis muscle. It is a vertical muscle that originates in the hairline. When it loses its tone and elasticity, it elongates by pushing into the eye brow muscles which then weakens the upper eye lids.

Your frontalis muscle can regain strength through isometric contraction exercise and this action lifts the forehead and the eye brows. By frequently exercising the muscles around the eyes and the forehead muscle horizontal lines will soften, the eye lids will open and the impaired vision? Well, in just a few weeks, your eye lids will lift and your eyes will look brighter. Try it! What do you have to lose – just saggy eye lids that make you look tired.

Rather than opting for temporary measures such as surgery and injections that may detrimentally alter the face, exercise will increase the distance between the eye brows and the eye lashes giving the user a lifted look. Your eyes will feel and look brighter and healthier without any risk, pain or recovery. Exercise works!

The Eyes Have It

After the age of 40, eye lids show signs of atrophy; in fact, the truth is that at 40, aging is affecting just more than eye lids. Eye brows are drooping and crows' feet are becoming apparent. The under eye is showing wear and tear too; deep lines, puffiness, hollowness are all glaring signs of aging.

The booming men and women of today know how important it is to be secure with the fact that we are who we are – souls of the world embracing all life has to offer.

This includes learning to be secure with who we are on the outside too. We want to be genuine, not superficial or plastic in our appearance and we want to put our best face forward so that we are recognized and complimented for our winning ways and self-confidence.

Looking in the mirror and seeing tired, hooded eyes, crows' feet and droopy eyebrows can send the normal person over the edge, dialing 911 for a plastic surgeon to remedy the situation. Oh sure, that's the "easy" way out. Surgery – cutting – scarring – pain – disappointment – pain – recovery time – pain – risk - infection – slow healing - and the list can go on and on. Surgery is not easy.

The media have been very proficient at keeping everyone abreast of the newest tricks (surgery/injections/strings) performed by plastic surgeons. The media have contributed to the $60 million plus spent on eye procedures in 2005; that's right, over 200,000 people shelled out $3,000 to $5,000 to plastic surgeons to temporarily lift the brow and tweak the upper and lower lids.

These costly, risky procedures can be replaced with exercise. That's right! Using one or two exercises can shorten, lift and tighten the very muscles doctors are cutting then suturing.

Surgery is temporary because even though the muscles have been cut and sutured into the desired position, they are going to continue to atrophy and elongate unless you exercise them. If you choose not to exercise the brows and forehead to maintain the surgical lift, you will soon see that another surgery is in your future.

Exercise is far superior to elective cosmetic eye surgery because there is no risk. Take risk, pain, bruising, blurred vision, big expense and disappointment out of the equation. Results begin immediately and continue daily as long as you spend 35 seconds a day exercising your brows and upper eyes.

Exercise is beneficial for everyone and what a terrific deterrent to looking old when you begin exercising your face before aging is apparent. Facial fitness is just as important as mental fitness, physical fitness and spiritual fitness.

Your face, the part of your body that resonates who you are is your power suit and when you look pretty and healthy, your confidence shows. Improving our appearance is age old and looking good impacts our daily lives whether we work at home or meet people daily through our life experiences. We know that when we feel good about ourselves, we are happier, more productive and life just seems easier.

Bottom line: If you look in the mirror and see a tired face looking back at you, just know that help is as close as your fingertips.

Facelift

Do It Yourself Facelift

Do you look great for your age? Do you look 10 years younger than you are? Do people constantly guess your age incorrectly? Are they shocked to find out your real age? How many years younger than your real age do people say you look? How does it make you feel to look so young?

What are your secrets to looking young? Is it your exercise, diet, clothes, hair, make-up or attitude?

Oprah has asked her viewers the above questions and it is curious to note that most people when they look closely at themselves in the mirror do not look younger than they did ten years ago, especially if they are over the age of fifty.

Why? Sagging facial muscles make you look older. Those hidden muscles situated beneath the skin begin to elongate as one ages. When this happens, the elongating muscles drag down the features, making your face look square rather than oval and all of a sudden, it is apparent that you have lost your youthful visage.

Using hair color, adopting a youthful attitude, wearing hip clothes and maintaining a youthful figure are certainly successful anti-aging tools. No matter how cleverly one uses these ploys, you cannot disguise an aging face.

Makeup and creams, lotions and potions will certainly mask fine lines and wrinkles. Today's cosmeceutical advances promise younger, softer looking skin but they can do nothing to lift jowls, pouches, hooded eyes, and a double chin.

Oh yes, there are injections and surgeries available for those risk takers who care little about the possible catastrophic consequences such as staph infection, disappointing results or even death.

The easy-breezy attitude of the medical profession mocks conventional wisdom that screams

"This is dangerous stuff!"

That's right – surgery is dangerous and should be used as the very last option. And those injections that plump and paralyze? Well, consider this: Do you really know and understand what is being injected into your body? Are the long-term health risks worth repeating several times per year, year after year?

Injections and surgeries are temporary at best because aging continues to affect the downward slide of the muscles.

Over the past few years a social stigma has arisen around aging. No longer is it acceptable to gracefully accept the lines, wrinkles, sags and bags. Aging is not what it used to be and people want to fight the look of old. We feel young on the inside and we want our faces and bodies to match. The new mantra is: Let's resist aging every step of the way!"

Does this mean that we all must meekly submit to injections and surgery? Can we turn back the hands of time without resorting to risk and the loss of our nest egg? Yes, we can and here is how: Specialized facial exercises will keep you looking younger than your years.

Consider this: most facial plastic surgeons tell their clients that a face lift will result in a reduction of five to ten years off one's appearance. Now this sounds enticing and easy, doesn't it? But, it's not. A surgical procedure takes months and months to heal. And, once you have allowed cutting on your face, you never, ever look like you. You have been forever altered.

Sometimes the results are startling and all you wanted was to look refreshed.

A Do It Yourself Facelift makes perfect sense. Not only is the process easy and reliable, there is no down time, no cutting, no drugs or IV's and most of all, no surprises. Risking your life and your beauty for the sake of looking younger is insane.

Facial exercise will help you rediscover the face you thought you had lost forever. This all natural process uses contraction and resistance of the muscles so they shorten and plump up. The action of using your thumbs and fingers in white cotton gloves nourishes the face with increased oxygenated blood and because the muscles are attached directly to the skin, you look refreshed and younger using these specialized techniques just minutes a day.

The dedication to facial exercise will undo the look of aging and you can do it yourself without ever harming your beautiful face.

So You Think You Need a Facelift

Looked in the mirror only to hypercritically proclaim: "I need a facelift!"? If so, you are not alone. Every person over the age of 40 has begun to see subtle shifting in their facial appearance. Out of nowhere lines and folds have begun their development and all of a sudden, the once tight, sculpted chin has slackened leaving you feeling pretty glum knowing that you are beginning to look older than you ever thought possible.

You also know that if you aren't somehow, someway proactive, this aging is not going to correct itself.

There are only a few methods that will return the look of youthfulness to your face; some are natural, some are painful and expensive and some are just ludicrous gimmicks that deplete you of funds and subject you to great risk and bodily harm.

Which one would you choose?

The most talked about anti-aging remedies are terribly risky and dangerous because long term results have not been determined or documented. This includes injections and surgery.

Injections of foreign substances and cadaver material will definitely change your appearance; lips become misshapen and if the injections are used in the face, the face looks plasticized and unnatural. In order to maintain the results, further injections are required to be repeated over and over again. Just how many substances can the body endure? No one knows.

Surgery is very risky as well – surgery is a crap shoot because no one can guarantee the results of a procedure. Not only are there scars that produce loss of sensation and feeling in the excised area, there is always a risk of infection and disappointment because the face is forever distorted by surgery. Further aging is accentuated because the muscles and skin are now draped unnaturally; the face loudly shouts that your surgical face lift needs refreshing.

One interesting item in the marketplace is the hand-held, battery powered, electro-stimulation device that shoots electrical micro-currents into the face. These devices can create a slight contraction of the muscle which may affect the skin very temporarily after four to six weeks of use; usually the user needs to continually treat the area each day to create and then maintain the results.

There are cautions that need to be heeded using these devices. Over-use is a common side effect that can cause permanent damage such as involuntary muscle twitching which is not attractive and can be very disturbing to witness. An annoying stinging sensation is another by-product of superficial stimulation to the epidermal layer. Without resistance, the results are very temporary.

Another consideration beyond price and risk regarding injections and surgeries are the qualifications of the person executing the procedure. Is this person a physician? Is this person a dentist or a gynecologist performing plastic surgery? What's a girl to do?

Use a zero risk, no side-effect solution. It's true; a proven technique does exist that can correct aging, sagging faces. This solution is fast, safe and totally amazing.

Highly specialized facial exercises can easily restore your face to its former youthfulness. These exercises are easy to learn and easy to perform. They do not cause wrinkles as some physicians would like you to believe, rather, these exercises lift your face so dramatically, the results rival a magic wand.

In hardly any time at all eyelids lift and fine lines and wrinkles smooth. Your cheeks become prominent as your jaw sculpts and firms. From day one of this type of facial retraining muscles and skin respond to increased oxygenation caused by contraction and resistance exercises. The muscles begin to plump up, shorten and lift. Your skin responds by following the new, youthful positioning of the facial muscles. In just weeks your face looks revitalized and younger.

Keep in mind you can safely alter the shape and contour of your face and neck without an invasive, expensive, painful or risky procedure. These dire consequences are totally unnecessary if beauty and youthfulness are your desire.

Imagine yourself looking as young as you feel and you made it happen using only your thumbs and fingertips.

Jowls

How to Disguise Jowls

Have you looked into the mirror only to discover that your face has begun to slip and slide in a downward direction and there's hanging skin dangling along your jaw? Well, that, according to Webster's Dictionary is the definition of a jowl.

You do not have to be overweight to see the slackening signs of age on your face; this slackening is due to atrophied facial muscles that pool into other muscles and muscle groups. Interestingly, the facial skin is attached directly to the facial muscles so when your facial muscles begin to lose their tone and vitality, you will notice that your skin begins to behave differently. You may begin to look drawn, tired and somewhat haggard.

The resemblance to an older family member might become apparent as you wonder just how in the world Aunt Hilda's jowls came to live on your face. This type of aging is not hereditary; rather, if you are over the age of twenty five, your once tight facial muscles are beginning to battle with Mother Nature. If you see jowls, you might also be saddened to see sagging eye lids and cheeks that no longer portray apples when you smile.

By now you have probably realized that jowls cannot be disguised using makeup or skin care items. No matter how sophisticated a product sounds or how promising the claims, jowls, pouches, the dreaded wattle and more are real signs of aging that need more than just topical applications. To rid your face rather of jowls and pouches, double chins, droopy foreheads, etc., requires deep muscle treatments using specialized facial exercises.

Of course, there are invasive modalities offered by some physicians that may have you running scared and you should! Cutting perfectly healthy tissue or injecting chemicals into areas that can easily affect the brain is not the easy answer to aging. If you opt for these types of unnatural fixes, you may find that the cookie cutter norm does not suit you. At first glance, you may look unrecognizable to your friends, family and co-workers and there is no camouflaging face work of this type

Aging that is propped up using injections with untested ingredients that plump and paralyze will not stop the downward slide of muscles and skin. Choosing surgery will not stop aging in your face either. The muscles and skin will continue to make their way "south;" your face may look misshapen after using these modes of treatment as hidden sutures coupled with the waning effects of injections take their toll on your once pristine face and before you know it, you might look and feel pretty discouraged with your appearance.

Rather than use costly, risky and scary methods that may not produce the desired effect, just know that by using safe, sane and tested natural methods can work quickly to lift, tone and tighten sagging facial features. Facial exercise, using your thumbs and fingers as age erasers, requires only minutes each day in front of a mirror. There is no pain, no back breaking outlay of cash and certainly no risk to your good health when you choose this natural method over injections and surgery.

The results are what count and with easy isometric movements, your results will be easily garnered and they are lasting results that will keep you looking substantially younger than your peers. You will hardly believe your eyes as your face begins rehabilitation; slowly at first using only two exercises for the upper eyes and upper cheeks. Week after week, when more exercises are added, your entire face and neck will lift and tighten. You can look 10 to 15 years younger in about 9 to 12 weeks.

Our small facial muscles weave over and under each other and attach to bone on one end in our hairline. Just as muscles in our bodies enjoy a workout, the muscles in our faces benefit from the oxygenated blood and the plumped up skin improvement is almost instantly apparent.

Mark Berman, MD, Santa Monica, CA, has studied facial exercise and has this to say, "I've seen the results and they're really quite impressive. And actually if you think about it, this makes sense medically. After all, when you exercise your body, you're going to tone and tighten the muscles in your body. So why not apply the same principles to your face? If you stay with the program, it should work indefinitely.

Whether you're 30 or 70, you're going to see a definite change... I've seen the results, and it works!"

Disguising jowls or rather reducing the appearance of jowls and other facial flaws caused by sagging muscles is possible using facial exercise only a few minutes each day. What do you have to lose? Only that tired looking face that keeps you looking old. Your appearance will greatly improve and your confidence will soar.

Lips

Full Lips Are Still Hot

Full, pouty, sensual lips are in the news. And it's all the same news; i.e. three young, hopeful women trying several topical items hoping they will see noticeable changes in the plumpness of their lips. In truth, the results are so temporary; the user will never experience any substantial lip pouting.

Lips are soft tissue; they easily lose hydration and shrink when men and women reach a certain age. The area surrounding the lips is muscle. As the orbicularis orris muscle shrinks due to atrophy and no exercise, the lips begin to implode. They appear smaller because they are affected by the collapse of the mouth muscle into the soft tissue.

After a while, the lips look dormant; they become thinner and usually lose their well-accentuated borders and contours. Likely, small lines will invade the area where the border was once prominent. Women see little lines that disturb their lipstick and liner; lip putties and topical preparations will slightly help to "fill in the cracks" but these are only temporary.

Many women and some men will try soft tissue augmentation to enhance their lips. There are many injected types of filler offered by physicians; these, too, are temporary and may cause discoloration, lopsidedness and swelling.

Some fillers are human derived (cadaver material!); some are animal and non-animal sources. These materials are "purified" before use then dehydrated, re-hydrated and then either injected or pulled through tunnels underneath the lip. Does that sound scary? These methods and modalities will have to be repeated over and over again for the user to maintain the enhancement.

So how does one enlarge the lips without pain, recovery time and expense? If you are serious about protecting your lips, your face, here is a proven exercise to give new life to your mouth:

While standing in front of a mirror, put the heels of both hands together. Place your thumbs in your mouth in a "V" position. Push the lip muscle outward without creating any lines around the mouth or lip area. The entire upper lip surface should be smooth and oval. Compress the upper lip muscles against your thumbs and hold for a count of five seconds. Remove your thumbs, take a deep breath, exhale and repeat the above movement for 10 seconds. Again, remove your thumbs, take a deep breath and exhale. Repeat the above movement twice for another twenty seconds.

Stand back and look at your face...keep it still and relaxed while you experience the rush of oxygenated blood and strength to your upper lip. Watch closely as your mouth corners turn upward...and your lips feel fuller, now marvel at the new, appealing you.

Fuller Lips – How Lip Enhancement Works

Aaaahhhhh, fuller, younger looking, pouty lips. Full lips are definitely a sign of "youth" but what happens to our lips when we begin to mature? Lips become thinner, less attractive and pretty soon, one just might give up wearing lipstick because the top lip virtually disappears, especially when smiling. When this shrinking act is apparent in the mirror, usually vertical lines begin to invade the lips making a mature women look positively ancient.

Women aren't the only ones who want softer, fuller lips. Men whose lips are thin and hard may portray a steely attitude in the boardroom; however, men with fuller lips look more attractive, boyish and younger.

Lips are soft tissue and as a man or woman begins to mature, volume dissipates which means tissue shrinks.

There are many modalities for revitalizing soft tissue in lips; the old standby - bovine collagen, Zyderm® and Zyplast® has competition. Restylane®, CosmoDerm® and ComoPlast® (human {cadaver} collagen), Radiance®, Artecoll® and others have entered the market of "fillers". These new fillers do not require skin testing for allergic reactions and they are all injected. The procedure time varies from 3-10 minutes and some patients relate that these types of injections can be painful. These services can be relatively expensive because they're not permanent fixes and these injections must be repeated every few months to maintain lip fullness. The most common side effect, as with any injection, is redness, bruising and swelling at the injection site that typically lasts less than three weeks.

A more permanent lip procedure that is widely used is Gortex. Strips of Gortex (threads of foam-like material) are inserted into the lips; the lips do become somewhat larger after the procedure is completed but some users complain that their lips feel hard, not soft and supple. Some of these implants cannot be removed if a problem arises because the lip tissue grows into and around the implant. Possible complications include infection, migration or extrusion of the implants and lip asymmetry is a concern.

Another somewhat permanent solution is fat injections; a patient's own fat is removed from usually the tummy or buttocks, washed and then re-injected into the lips. While this is probably a fairly safe modality, the fat tends to reabsorb rather quickly, deflating the lips.

Recently over the counter glosses, lipsticks, and other types of topical preparations have been introduced promising fuller, poutier lips with more definition and volume. Many cosmetic companies have jumped on this bandwagon promising the users that their special ingredients will produce full, luscious lips after a few weeks of use. In fact, there have been over 200 new products introduced to the marketplace in the last two years ranging in price from $6.99 to almost $40. Instead of traffic stopping lips, some of these topical products have produced burns, mouth sores and empty pockets.

Some cosmetic companies do use natural components in their formulas but some of the formulas may be misleading. No product can deliver the look of a collagen injection in a topical. How these products work is through the use of an irritating ingredient such as niacin, cinnamon, caffeine or peppermint; these ingredients may cause some temporary swelling via dilation of the blood vessels along with mild inflammation, giving the illusion of fullness. Some preparations require the user to rub the lips briskly for several minutes and this friction results in some degree of temporary swelling.

Many women and men want fuller lips because poutier lips make them feel sexier and more alluring. Consumers are willing to spend a lot of money to have "the look"; but not everyone agrees that the topicals deliver what they have promised. Dr. Sam Most, Chief of Facial Plastic and Reconstructive Surgery at the University of Washington in Seattle asked seven women to use a certain topical whose website says their product increases actual lip volume and contour an average of 40.7 percent; Dr. Most said, "In subjects who used the product as directed over a long term there was no visible change in the lips."

Is there an actual difference in using topical applications that promise full, pouty lips or is lipstick and a liner enough? Maybe Yoki Ono, a saleswoman at a Madison Avenue designer boutique, quoted in the NY Times, has the answer: "You might as well get some extra-spicy Buffalo wings and eat them."

Or better yet, save yourself a bundle of cash and brush your lips with a baby's toothbrush and petroleum jelly.

Will Fuller Lips Make Your Face Look Younger?

If you have smiled at yourself in the mirror or meticulously pored over recent photos trying to decide just what is different about your facial appearance, consider this: Lips shrink with age and if your smile is showing more teeth than you remember, your lips need a tune-up.

The beauty barons have certainly jumped on the proverbial band wagon because we see ads for lip enhancement product advertisements in the drug stores, on TV, magazines, web pages, e-zines and more. The choices are astounding and you just might be confused by all the hype to create fuller lips.

Years ago when you realized that your lips were not quite as full as they were when you were in your early years, you may have pulled a Joan Crawford; drawing outside the line was fairly popular for awhile. Maybe you fooled most of the people but you knew that your lips did not have a pout and you probably looked a little funny.

In the 80's and 90's plastic surgeons began to experiment with certain fillers that were either injected or implanted surgically to enlarge mostly the top lip. These temporary fixes transformed the lips but the results were not always optimal. The lips sometimes felt very hard, rock-like, and those lumps and bumps shouted to everyone that your lips were less than authentic.

Using unnatural substances and chemicals to plump up your lips means that you are willing to spend a lot of money and to risk damaging the very essence of who you are.

Lip Serums and Potions came on the scene and they have been snatched up by women on most every continent. Buyer beware because even those innocent and sometimes very expensive, gooey lip preparations that promise to enlarge your lips may subject you to a very nasty surprise, especially if you are sensitive to certain chemicals and ingredients.

Do they really deliver on their promises to make your lips fuller? Or do they just provide a sensation that something is happening?

Why is lip enhancement important? What causes lips to lose their fullness? Lip and eyes are focal points on our faces. If the lips appear thin and hard, this affects the entire face. Typically, women stop wearing lipstick because of bleed lines surrounding their lips. Lines begin to form above the lips and around the mouth when there is less fullness.

Lip tissue is soft tissue. This provides fullness and definition to our lips. When lips lose definition and shape, our mouths can look withered and drawn, even misshapen.

Muscle atrophy is partly to blame. If your top lip is shrinking the muscle surrounding the lips is losing its battle with Mother Nature. Maybe you have pursed your lips, maybe you need a better bite or maybe you just need to pump up those lips.

There is a safe and sane lip product that will create full, pouty, more kissable lips without lumps, bumps or risks. Rather than injections or surgery or anything gooey that burns, sears delicate tissue or creates mouth sores you might want to try a lip pump device.

A lip pump device creates a very gentle vacuum action that slowly coaxes your own body fluid into the lip area and locks it there so that the size of the lips increases about fifty percent. Daily use assures that your lips stay fuller longer and longer.

This natural process of lip enhancement does not put anything into the body. There is no pain and there are no drawbacks. Oh sure there has been some reported bruising for those over zealous users but basically it's a safe bet that if you would like to see fuller, younger looking lips, the lip pump will work for you.

The process of creating full, Luscious Lips does not happen overnight; rather, one must first condition the lips by slowing using the pump for just seconds per day. Using the pump for five two-second pulls for the first two weeks ensures that the lips establish and maintain fullness. After the initial two week conditioning period, the user can then use the device up to 120 seconds per day.

The lip pump is affordably priced, there is no risk and it can be used by both men and women. Results are a small miracle especially for those whose lips are without definition, color and fullness.

Look Younger

Divorce Makes You Look Older, While Facial Exercise Lifts Your Face

Margie thought her marriage would last forever; whenever she heard or read statistics concerning divorce, she brushed them aside never believing for one moment that she would ever find her husband boring or inattentive to the point that she would even consider divorce, let alone become a divorcee. Over the years Margie noticed she smiled less and less, her eyes no longer held a twinkle and the level of fun in her life greatly subsided. Oh sure, she had special times with her grandchildren, her girlfriends and her children but she noticed she had long felt bored, indifferent with life in general and even restless toward her husband.

Realizing that she could easily give up on their once very meaningful relationship, she knew the word "divorce" could indeed become a reality. Could she handle living life on her own?

Divorce, according to the Holmes-Rahe Scale, is the second most stress filled life event, just shy of losing a prized possession such as a child or a spouse.

Separation can mean loss of job, the end of a friendship, the failure of a relationship. Sometimes emotional trauma can turn our smiles upside down as we wear the look of sadness and separation on our faces. Divorce, death, disappointment and other feelings that harbor resentment, anger and bitterness can age us quickly.

Unfortunately this is a type of mental programming that produces physical displays such as down turned mouths, tired looking eyes, a lack of radiance and even illness. Our bruised psyche and emotions are typically visible in our faces. Witness a long-time girlfriend showing up for lunch, down in the mouth and mad as heck - we see her frustration on her face as we query, "What's up with you?!?"

Sometimes women give up when they experience loss and defeat; there are some women who live like there is no failure.

Which one are you?

Getting on track again is the goal when you are ready for change. Change your thinking, change your life. If you allow fear to keep you stuck in an unhappy, dismal place this, too, can age our faces quickly. Couple fear and vulnerability with antidepressants that are typically prescribed when one is feeling blue and you have the recipe for an old looking appearance.

Living life on purpose using facial exercise breaks the ice around your heart.

Face work, mirror work, positive thoughts and affirmations can change your attitude and the shape and contour of your face.

Yes, facial plastic surgery and injections that plump and paralyze are easily accessible avenues if you are looking old and tired but remember these avenues have consequences. Some of them can be dire.

It is in your best interest for optimum health and fiscal responsibility that makes facial exercise so attractive. Using only your thumbs and fingers in white cotton gloves while facing your mirror, you quickly see results that demonstrate how easy it is to maintain your face with simple exercise movements.

It is no secret that using extraneous modalities can certainly make you look different but even injections can make you look overdone, even matronly.

Surely you have seen celebrity faces that have been shot full of chemicals that were intended to plump up lines and wrinkles and instead of seeing a youthful face, a full face appears that is devoid of natural contour.

Paralyzing injections also have their drawbacks; watching an actress's immobile face is one thing but seeing a face whose forehead does not move or eyes that no longer portray expression, live and in person is very telling. Add nips 'n' tucks and you have the recipe for a misshapen, hardly recognizable face.

Most treatments are expensive, temporary and only mask facial aging symptoms. Injections, surgery, laser treatments, facials and peels and electro-stimulation devices do not address the underlying cause of aging in your face.

Facial exercise gets to the root cause of saggy skin and droopy facial features. Facial muscles support the skin and when they are exercised skin becomes radiant and flushed with oxygenated blood. The fingers and thumbs anchor tiny muscles so that they can tighten and lift.

Looking healthy, looking your best doesn't have to involve risk, pain or a lot of money. You can take control of your face without cutting or suturing or injecting any foreign substances that might have long-term side effects when you choose muscle retraining movements.

Imagine that you look ten to fifteen years younger, portraying a prettier, lifted face without the hassle of time away from friends and family, the risk of infection or other horrors or even the embarrassment of a botched procedure.

Using natural facial rehabilitation methods boosts your confidence because you are in charge. You won't have to worry about breaking the bank or putting your beautiful face in harm's way.

Feeling good about you no matter if there is a significant other in the picture or not is the priceless payoff.

Exercise Your Face to Look Healthier & Younger

Do you have a problem area on your face that you would like to change? Double chin, droopy eyes, jowls, pouches, crow's feet or marionette lines? Aging is as sneaky as sun damage and it seems that in a twinkling of an eye, your face can look so different that you might wonder just who is that person staring back at you in the mirror?

Could facial exercise be the answer to the age old question −"Can I maintain a youthful appearance?" Must I spend my children's inheritance to stave off Mother Nature's footprints across my face?

You can certainly turn back the clock with facial exercise that employs resistance and isometric contractions of the muscles using the thumbs and fingers. This doesn't mean that you will look sixteen or even twenty again but shaving off ten or fifteen years from your appearance with exercise rivals the results of most plastic surgery procedures.

Plastic surgery techniques do not stop the aging process; muscles in the face continue to make their downward slide dragging the skin unnaturally, creating the need for more and more surgical procedures. With exercise, the muscles become stronger, the skin looks revitalized and lifted. Most importantly, facial exercises can be performed inexpensively at home.

The muscles of the face elongate just like the muscles in your arms, thighs and buttocks; in fact, the muscles in the face will have elongated about one-half inch by the time most people have reached the age of 55. The elongation is the result of atrophy of the muscles and gravity. Even though we talk, sing or laugh, the muscles continue to soften and become lax; it's only when the facial muscles are specifically exercised do they begin to plump up and support your skin better.

The elongation of facial muscles affects every area of your face. For instance, the "apples" in your upper cheeks may not be positioned prominently, in fact, when a smile is made, rather than seeing fullness high on the cheeks, the muscles may appear flat and midway between the nose and mouth.

If you add one-half inch to the length of your forehead, your eye area suffers because the downward motion compresses into the brows. What happens if you add one-half inch or more to the area under the chin? The dreaded wattle is developing. One-half inch added to the jaw line means jowls are forming.

Beginning a facial exercise program to sculpt and contour the face may seem daunting at first because the movements and positioning feel somewhat awkward. Remember when you first learned to ride a bicycle? It was so scary! But after a few days of lumps and bumps, you were pedaling like you were a pro. It's the same with facial exercise, once you become familiar with the movements, you will marvel that these simple steps can easily produce a younger looking face.

You will want to take beginning photos before you start a facial exercise regimen so that you can track your progress and you will want to update your photos at the end of every third week. In about three weeks friends and colleagues will begin noticing that something is definitely different about you. They may think you have changed your hair in some way or that you are sleeping better but you will know what they're seeing is your pretty face returning.

In hardly any time at all, you will notice how smooth and refreshed your skin looks; your face glows with radiance from increased oxygenation to the muscles and those sagging, droopy muscles are now portraying a more youthful looking you. Without surgery, drugs or anything harmful you can turn back the clock and look at least 10-15 years younger.

Facial Exercise - The Sensible, Practical Solution to Looking Younger

Medical experts recently released a warning that only healthy people should be allowed to have cosmetic and plastic surgery. DUH!

Serious complications from cosmetic surgery procedures have been speculated about for years. The untimely death of Donda West, mother of rap artist Kanye West, who wanted several procedures performed - one right after the other while she lie oblivious to her impending death due to several health issues she evidently ignored - has spiked more interest in the pitfalls of surgery.

Surgery is risky business.

The latest issue of the Plastic and Reconstructive Surgery Journal disclosed that one in every 298 patients who had a cosmetic procedure suffered serious complications, with one death recorded in every 51,459 cases.

What is deemed a "serious complication"? Bleeding, excessive vomiting, bruising, respiratory and heart problems are the top five complications from breast augmentation, face lift, liposuction and tummy tucks. Serious complications from anesthesia can also include loss of memory and cognitive functions - postoperative cognitive dysfunction (POCD).

A lot of Baby Boomers have health challenges: Diabetes, heart disease, high blood pressure and more are prevalent in those men and women born after 1946. Lots of prescriptions are written for them and that poses yet another health risk as many people ingest between five and twenty-five medications per day.

Surgery + prescription drugs + ailments = DISASTER!

Injections to plump and paralyze sagging, droopy facial features can have their pitfalls, too. The number one concern is that injections are temporary and must be repeatedly used over and over each and every year that a person wants to look younger . Keep in mind that these new drugs have had no long term testing.

How can one person's face be subjected to many, many injections for years and years? How many surgeries can the face endure? Is there a saturation point?

When you think about it, a younger looking face looks healthy. Sometimes surgery and injections miss the mark with their unmistakable tell-tale signs of use and overuse.

We can disguise our bodies with clothing. And we can disguise aging in the face without using substances or procedures.

That's right. Without drugs, surgery or injections, specialized facial exercises can help your face look lifted and tighter.

Right now you can begin to lift those droopy eyelids that develop as our eyebrows drop using simple resistance and contraction movements. Even those pesky jowls and pouches can become less evident when your cheeks lift, smoothing and flattening the nose to mouth lines.

Exercise for your body produces a toned, sleek look. The same type of resistance and contraction movements will help your face look refreshed, lifted and younger. Using your "age erasers", your fingers and thumbs in white cotton exercise gloves, you can begin to systematically strengthen and tone your facial muscles.

These easy to follow movements can be completed in just minutes a day in the privacy of your home.

What results can you expect and how long before you see them? Most users of this type of exercise program see results almost immediately. Until your muscles become stronger, the new look will slowly develop but once your muscles are in better shape, you will notice that you look and feel differently when you look in the mirror.

Your peers will also begin to realize there is something going on with your look. They will wonder if you have changed your hairstyle. Maybe they will think you've been getting some really good rest or that your new diet has made you look refreshed and invigorated.

After some weeks, they may even approach you only to ask if you have had recent face work as they look for scars and seams. Your new face will be the envy of your friends and most likely you will look substantially younger than you have in years when you choose facial exercise.

Safe, natural, no surprises; facial exercise is the smart solution!

If You Look Younger You Might Live Longer

It is not surprising to learn that Danish scientist's say that looking young may mean that you live a younger life. This study, published online in the British Medical Journal, suggests that people who look younger may also live longer.

Now why do you think this is possible?

Is it because when you take steps every day to maintain and even improve your health that it shows on your face? Probably.

Consider the average upbringing; in these times with usually both parents working full-time jobs, some children may be introduced to pre-packaged foods, GMO or irradiated foods and water that is full of chlorine and fluoride from birth. These children, hopefully, will grow to understand the need to eat healthy, organic fruits and vegetables and use only purified water that removes chemicals that over time can sap our good health.

Children who regularly exercise usually fare better than those who are raised without exercise. Obesity levels are lower, they sleep better, their cognitive skills are improved and the list of benefits goes on and on.

Exercise is not just for kids. As adults mature exercise is important because it helps us to maintain our strength, our weight, our balance and the health of our heart, lungs and total being. Exercise is the fountain of youth and when you add nutrition to the mix, you provide an environment to thrive.

So, the question is: "Are you thriving?"

When the Danish scientists followed their test subjects to determine how perceived age correlates with survival, their peers viewed 1800 photographs of 387 sets of twins (352 men and 422 women) that were measured by who appeared more youthful along with physical and cognitive functioning. Turns out that the participants could blame their wrinkles, brown spots, red spots, dilated blood vessels on the very things that directly attribute to aging - sun, smoking, weight issues, alcohol and chemical indulgence plus sagging facial muscles.

All of us carry genetic factors that influence the condition and appearance of our skin. Perhaps we look at our older siblings and perceive that they look younger; maybe they've had less stress, maybe they have regularly exercised and taken better care of their heath.

And, maybe they have used facial exercise as their best kept anti-aging secret.

That's right! Facial exercise can help a face look 10-15 years younger without using anything invasive. It works for men and women, the process hardly takes any time at all. You're never too young or too old to begin a regimen of exercise that will lift, tone and tighten sagging facial muscles.

Just as exercise is the fountain of youth for your body, facial exercise that uses resistance and contraction can act as 'the fountain' for your face.

The stress reducing movements change the shape and contour of your face using techniques that can be completed in just minutes a day. You will feel and see the differences daily and your friends and family will marvel at the renewed vitality they see in your face.

Most users proclaim they look years younger after learning facial exercise; some say that look 10-15 years younger. Imagine, using exercise instead of surgery and injections to keep you looking younger.

Bottom line: if your face looks old, you cannot blame your genes because the secret to youth begins with tiny, baby steps such as not smoking, watching your weight, eating healthy, organic foods, policing drug and alcohol use and certainly watching how much time you spend in the sun.

Environmental damage happens both inside and on the outside of our bodies. Protection comes in many forms such as supplement use, the products we use on our bodies, the water we drink and even the thoughts we think.

The scientists are right - if you look younger, you most likely will live longer. Looking younger is all about how you portray your calling card - your body!

Look Years Younger in Just Minutes!

Women's magazines and certain home pages for major search engines typically relay the latest and greatest five ways to stop aging now, seven helpful tips to stop unwanted hair growth and even ten ways to leave your lover. If you are like most people, these headlines draw you into reading or at least skimming the article to see if any of these tips resonate with your life needs.

Some of these tips are meant to tickle your funny bone but when dispensing sage advice, they just might miss the mark.

A recent magazine and internet article offered information regarding under eye circles, boosting your eyebrows and using under eye concealers.

"Give Crow's Feet the Boot" stated that these lines are formed as a result of lost collagen in the skin and gave the impression that by using a topical retinol or Vitamin A derivative, those lines and wrinkles would be lessened.

Yes, loss of collagen can certainly create lines and wrinkles but most Crow's feet are caused by repeated squinting motions coupled with an elongated forehead muscle that has pooled into the eyebrow muscles. Using a topical treatment to treat this type of compression may very temporarily ease the look of Crow's Feet but when squinting is repeated and gravity sets in, the lines and creases will return.

Using chilled eye compresses to temporarily alleviate under eye puffiness caused by fluid retention is well known; however, did you know that by decreasing your salt intake and slightly increasing your water consumption can deflate those puffy eyes?

In addition, try sleeping on a higher, firmer pillow and slide a one-inch book under each leg of your bed's headboard to slightly incline the pitch so that you are not sleeping flat. Check with your Doc if you are taking medication and under eye puffiness persists because long-term puffiness may indicate another condition.

Lifting your eyebrows by reshaping your eyebrow's arch or stenciling doesn't really create a difference if your eye lids are flabby, lined and moving toward your lashes. Hooded eye lids are a result of the eyebrow muscle losing its tone and resiliency; plucking or drawing does not correct the problem.

What makes a difference to help you look years younger? Can circles, droopy eyelids, brows and other age related appearances be remedied?

The best kept anti-aging secret is facial exercise! Facial exercise can stop crow's feet, lift sagging eyelids, lighten and brighten the under eye area and much, much more.

Concerned that your under eye bags are there forever and those dark circles make you look like a zombie even though you daily use a concealer in every conceivable shade?

Here is a movement you can begin to help you look years younger in just seconds a day.

Try the 100-circle exercise for under eye puffiness and dark circles: Apply a very small amount of an eye treatment product to the ring finger of your dominant hand. Begin under the inner brow and lightly trace upwards and outwards until a full circle has been completed around the upper and lower eye region. Gently perform this exercise about 100 times around each eye making certain the under eye area is well lubricated before you begin.

You can stop the formation of Crow's feet by elevating the forehead and upper eye brows. Prove this now: place the three middle fingers of each hand underneath your eye brows and push them upward. Do you see how the Crow's feet are no longer apparent?

Simple resistance exercise can change the shape and contour of your face quickly without risk or harm. In just minutes a day, your face can look revitalized and fresh naturally.

Crow's feet and sagging eyebrows can be remedied by performing one exercise that requires only 35 seconds of your time each day.

Enjoy the confidence knowing that your face can be saved without resorting to silly tactics that might disappoint you.

Looking Younger – The Commitment

The Baby Boomers always knew they would look younger and indeed they have. Whoever coined the phrase "Sixty is the New Forty" certainly must have been a Baby Boomer who grew up defying anything that reeked of old.

We promised ourselves that we would never look like our parents or act like them. We adopted the unspoken rule of 'tie dye forever' and 'down with the establishment'.

Little did we know that the establishment would snare us, rope us into believing that we need to cut our bodies and invade our systems with toxins and poisons – all in the name of beauty?

Somehow we were sold out. In the sixties and seventies, even into the eighties and nineties that pact we had made to always look and act young was eroded by an industry that promised beauty at the end of a syringe and a scalpel.

This type of self improvement has rapidly become a type of self mutilation. In the name of beauty more and more men and women are allowing their perfectly healthy faces to be altered with methods that may not produce the desired results and these modalities can certainly jeopardize one's health and well being.

Somehow a misconception has been plied that surgery and injections are easy routes to erase the years; it is not.

Remember seeing "The Swan" and "Extreme Makeover?" Most of us were wowed with the results of plastic surgery and dentistry that were paraded before us. The contestants did not see themselves for six weeks so imagine their surprise at their unveiling. New faces, sculpted bodies, bigger breasts, hair styling and more were in evidence with every contestant.

Some of the contestants endured up to seventeen procedures in a six week period of time; were the results as pleasant as the show producers wanted us to believe?

Not always. Here is how one contestant reflected on her surgeries that were fraught with complications: "Cosmetic surgery is "only a quick fix. ... When you come back to reality, you're still you," said Lorrie Arias, Corona, CA.

After multiple procedures was she happier, more beautiful and confident in her new appearance. No.

Lorrie is basically a recluse now and she regrets her decision to participate in the makeover show. She cautions those thinking of using plastic surgery by saying that she doesn't believe her new look was worth the cost because she continues to suffer from a botched thigh lift that left her once beautiful skin with a dented, sunken hole. In addition Arias says that when she touches her eyebrows she feels it on the back of her scalp and her belly is numb. She can no longer comfortably tip her head back.

Lorrie Arias is not alone.

Does she need revision surgery? Probably but who pays?

Procedures can go terribly wrong and if emotional and psychological baggage is mixed with self esteem issues and hidden health challenges, this might be the recipe for disaster.

Body dysmorphic disorder (BDD) is a chronic condition defined as someone excessively concerned with their physical features.

Maybe you wonder if you or your friends might have a tendency toward self-loathing your appearance. If you frequently eye yourself with disdain you might fall prey to the hype of injections and surgery.

Perhaps you've seen friends start with paralyzing injections then move onto injections that plump, maybe a nose job is next and then certainly liposuction and thermage. After that more injections, laser treatments and an eye lift.

Maybe BDD is a result of too many consultations with plastic surgeons that destroy any confidence you have in your appearance with recommendations for many procedures.

Maintaining a youthful look without using extraneous means takes a commitment to love and care for you without resorting to invasive procedures like surgery and injections.

Using exercise is a loving way to care for your face and it is one very effective treatment for an aging face. Just as your body appreciates the rush of oxygenated blood throughout the limbs and torso, your face will absolutely benefit from the nutrients and plumping provided by simple isometric exercise.

Using facial exercise rather than invasive procedures means you will age spectacularly without any danger, risk of infections or disappointment and no recovery time.

Looking younger just got easier!

Looking Younger is an Inside Job

Maintaining a positive mindset is a key to staving off the aging process. There are many techniques that can boost your positive mental attitude and help you age gracefully.

The awareness of who we are and where we want to go in life develops in your mind; you have control of every thought, action and deed. When one recognizes mind-power, life can become richer, easier and more fulfilling because you are cognizant of your energy, your thinking.

One avenue of awareness is through affirmations; these simple positive statements, steeped in belief that you are the master of your destiny, can help overcome many fears and doubts one may harbor. Tony Robbins, noted author and speaker, has a favorite that he repeats 500 times a day while jogging: "God's wealth is circulating in me. His wealth flows to me in avalanches of abundance. All my needs, desires and goals are met instantaneously for I am one with God and God is everything." Those are powerful words. Repeating these powerful, faith filled words many times a day will permeate your subconscious mind and soon you will find yourself repeating them over and over again each day.

Recently, NBC Today Show featured Katie Couric, Christy Brinkley and Cheryl Tiegs discussing how age and aging was being redefined; they concluded that age fifty is now the new thirty; age sixty is now the new forty. This redefinition of aging is possible because we look and act differently than our ancestors; we have transformed physically and mentally and most of us would like to think we're getting better at life.

Just think back 100 years, our life expectancy was approximately 47 years and now the average age of first time grandparents is 47.

Transformation of the self - awareness, actualization, comes from the inside. Many people believe if they are showing outward signs of aging, Botox or a visit to a plastic surgeon will give them the needed boost of self-confidence, sex appeal or happiness that is lacking in their lives. Once those procedures are done, some patients may be disappointed that their life did not magically transform: yes, the outside has been changed yet they may still feel empty and unfilled.

As life expectancy increases more and more anti-aging creams, pills and injections will be marketed to the baby boomers and zoomers. As it is today, we are inundated with lotions and potions that promote empty promises which mean there are a lot of disappointed people who have spent countless thousands of dollars chasing after the fountain of youth. Celebrities and models have set an unreachable goal for many as their airbrushed and retouched photos are splashed across beauty magazines, movie posters and billboards. They just look so perfect – no wrinkles, no bulging thighs or stomach that jiggles and gorgeous hair perfectly coifed.

Almost every emotion shows on our face – pain, joy, anger, stress, disappointment, frustration, sorrow, illness, hopelessness and love. When life happens the face becomes drawn and tired. At this point, some may seek professional help – plastic surgery. After a few nips and tucks, the newly altered face begins to loosen and aging becomes apparent again because surgical procedures or injections do not stop or reverse aging in the face.

What if you want to look and feel healthier and happier without going to extremes or spending a lot of money? Well, you can!

The true beauty of every person begins inside; it's an ongoing process of evolving emotions, understanding unconditional love and loving your self more. Happiness and health is achieved when we learn to treat each other with love, respect and honor; everyone benefits from our presence - our families, our friendships, our co-workers and each person we meet and greet.

A reliable alternative to facial injections and elective surgeries is facial exercise.

There is an internal change that occurs when you face yourself in the mirror and perform movements to correct an aging face; that change is self acceptance. As you learn to love your 'total' self, you will more and more appreciate that person in the mirror.

Will Looking Younger Help You Keep Your Job? Try Facial Exercise!

Facial plastic surgery does not boost your career.

Brains, desire for achievement, willingness to succeed as well as looking young, healthy, serene and fresh boosts your career.

Career advancement has long been linked to owning a handsome or pretty face; it is well documented that if you are one of those people who make the bigger strides in today's business climate, you probably are above average looking and stand over 5'9" tall.

The face matters.

Ever look in the mirror and see how age is affecting your face? Does it show the ravages of time, disappointment, stress and tiredness? Could this look affect your job performance and how people view your ideas?

Of course it does!

Looking fit, hearty and able-bodied goes a long way to shape your self-confidence as well as your image. Remaining competitive in the workplace requires that you take care of yourself; this means relearning dietary habits if you've been a junk food junkie, working out regularly to maintain or create a slimmer physique and learning a facial exercise routine that keeps your face in much better shape.

Just as you exercise your body in the gym with Pilates, yoga, aerobics and weight training, you can apply the same principles to retrain your facial muscles.

This means you can use facial exercise to substantially correct flaws like hooded eyes, sagging cheeks, jowls, pouches, the dreaded wattle and more, making facial plastic surgery unnecessary if your goal is to look 10-15 years younger.

You may wonder why this successful aging technique has been discounted, maligned, pooh-poohed and buried. Perhaps it is because a discovery like this, a facelift without surgery, drugs, sutures, pain, risk, disfigurement, injections, strings or electricity, could put the drug companies and docs out of business almost overnight.

You see, something natural, something that doesn't require intervention or administration by a physician or medical professional may seem too good to be true; after all, we have brainwashed via countless articles, advertisements and flyers to believe that surgery and injections will provide us with a new face - one that will transform our image and confidence as we navigate the ladder of success.

Choosing surgery and injections over a natural regimen such as facial exercise may not provide the results you are seeking. Even though surgical strides have greatly improved over the last one hundred years, they are not fool-proof and there are tremendous risks and complications that prevail.

The American Society of Plastic Surgeons discloses that eye lid surgery is the fourth most common surgical procedure. The average cost for eye lid surgery, cutting both eye lids, excising the extraneous tissue and then suturing the lids runs about $3500.

Scheduling and paying for surgery is the easy part but recuperation is another story. There are pitfalls and risks with every cosmetic and plastic procedure.

Do not be confused; exercise is natural and safe while surgery and injections always carry a degree of risk. There are no risks using exercise.

Looking ten years younger is the goal for most plastic procedures although we have all seen procedures on celebrities and others that fell short of helping the patient look younger, rather all that was accomplished was that it was evident that something was altered and it isn't exactly working.

Surgically altered eye lids can look misshapen, they may tear uncontrollably for a long time and they may appear red and irritated.

Eye lid surgery does not stop the forehead from lengthening. Eye lid surgery is temporary. As the forehead muscle weakens and elongates due to atrophy, this downward motion affects the distance between the eye brows and the eyelashes so it's quite possible that revision surgery will be recommended in a few years as the eyelids again begin to hood.

Learning and using exercise to strengthen your forehead and lift your eye brows puts you in the driver's seat. In hardly anytime at all, you will see results as the forehead tightens and the eye brows lift.

Isolating the muscles and muscle groups throughout the face then applying the resistance techniques will sculpt and contour, lift and tighten sagging facial muscles that create the look of old.

Using exercise means there are no mistakes, no tell-tale sutures, no recovery times, no big dollars out of pocket and no risk to your good health. Using exercise means you look refreshed, toned and healthy with a face that looks 5-10-even 15 years younger!

Your career advancement is firmly in your grasp with an all natural, no risk, inexpensive yet priceless technique that keeps you looking younger.

We Must Remain Cute at All Times

Oh, the perils men and women confront when they decide to allow cutting, injecting and even lasers on their beautiful, pristine, unspoiled faces.

Once a face is injected with chemical substances it is forever changed. Same with deciding to lop off sagging skin; no matter how experienced the surgeon, the once untouched face will forever display signs of alteration. Even laser treatments have proven to be iffy at best with unexpected burns and holes on chins and around the eyes when over aggressive actions are used.

Disguising aging is big business these days; not only are the docs vying for your dollars, the department stores, spas of every kind, drugstores and internet sites want you to buy their hyped anti-aging lotions, potions and serums.

We have been deluged with all sorts of anti-aging concoctions from the foreskin of baby penises to a rooster comb to specially bred fish that are willing to eat away at dead skin. EW! Do these preparations deliver on their promises or are they just clever advertisements that provoke wishful thinking.

Most people do not want to look old and the advertisers know this. Do they prey upon gullible, unsuspecting consumers who wish to look years younger? It is highly possible considering the multi-billion dollar industry of beauty. Just open any woman's magazine and beauty ads spill from the pages - perfume, jewelry, clothing, boots, hats, belts and of course, skin care and cosmetic procedures are given top billing.

Most aging in the face is a result of sagging facial muscles due to loss of muscle mass and sun damage so using just skin care alone cannot adequately alter your appearance. You must use something deeper than just topical skincare preparations if you desire a newer, fresher visage.

What you do on a daily basis also impacts the health and well being of your face.

Do you smoke? Is your diet void of fresh vegetables and fruit? What anti-aging activities do you participate in? Do you walk or engage in physical activity daily? Are you willing to initiate changes to help your body look and feel as young as you want it to?

Are you searching for the Fountain of Youth in all the wrong places?

Truly, the Fountain of Youth begins with exercise - facial exercise!

Facial exercise consists of small steps taken daily and these small steps lead you to a younger looking face without using drastic measures that puts your health at risk.

In just minutes a day you can create a more youthful face using your thumbs and fingers performing special exercises that act as your age erasers. You will not have to think about using extraneous, dangerous, painful modalities that are unreliable.

How can facial exercise stop an aging face? Can you really look years younger using a non-surgical method? What about those drooping eyes and sagging cheeks and that wayward chin? Can this type of aging be helped?

Without a doubt and here's why: Just like the muscles elongate in our arms, tummy, waist, thighs and hips when we do not maintain them adequately with exercise, our facial muscles can become out of shape as well. Now, we can camouflage and conceal sagging body muscles with body contouring lingerie, long black, flowing blouses and black, roomy slacks but hiding a double chin, deep nasal labial folds and hooded eye lids is impossible.

Here's why aging in our faces is so visible: our facial muscles weave over and under each other then attach to bone on one end; when they elongate from disuse or atrophy, they pool into other muscles and muscle groups. This action can create lines, wrinkles and folds that skin care cannot fix. Oh sure, there are lotions and potions that can soften the look of aging but to stop sagging facial muscles, error proof methods are required and it's not about surgery or injections that plump and paralyze.

In our faces, the muscles are attached directly to our skin so when we employ lifting and tightening exercises, the muscles respond and reposition and so does our skin. Our skin and muscles can lift back and up into the hairline so that sagging is minimized.

Yes, using facial exercise is a do it yourself facelift. Just like exercise works for our body, facial exercise can help turn back the clock so that your face can look five, ten even fifteen years younger in hardly any time at all.

How exciting to know that you can remain cute and pretty at all times without spending your children's inheritance. Love your face with exercise.

Men

Facial Exercise Keeps Men Handsome

Men of the twenty first century have certainly transformed their regard for personal upkeep. Gone is the Neanderthal thinking as most of them have no problem having their hair and nails professionally cared for and a lot of them have discovered facials, waxing and more that add to their good looks.

Yes, men of this new millennium have decided that they, too, want to keep Father Time at a distance. Just as women have proclaimed that 60 is the new 40, it hasn't taken long for men to adopt that same proclamation for themselves.

After all, looking as young as you feel is a very nice place to be.

Unfortunately, men's faces elongate and look older just like women's faces do. No matter how many creams, lotions and potions they use, facial muscles that are soft make even the most handsome man look older.

Jowls form along the jaw, eyes become hooded and tired looking and all of a sudden that once taut chin has become a real concern. These signs of aging are worrisome and you can expect that your facial muscles will elongate about one-half inch by your mid-fifties.

It is not surprising that some men have begun to explore certain cosmetic products such as eye treatments and masks and now they are beginning to use plastic procedures such as injections that plump and paralyze.

Some of these users have determined that the "paralyzed look" doesn't really suit them because it hampers their success quotient. How? The passive, no expression-look in the boardroom has its distractions; in fact, the no expression look could be dubbed the "powerless look".

Most men who have had face work done cannot disguise the tell-tale look of pulled skin, out of place suture lines and a skewed hairline that doesn't quite look natural. We've seen this look on celebrities who can afford the very finest care. Funny thing though, plastic and cosmetic surgeons cannot guarantee their work. That's right - you don't like the results - well, too bad.

The effects of temporary fixes like injections will eventually wear off but surgery is permanent but only temporarily permanent because the muscles that support the skin continue their downward slide affecting the skin in an unnatural way. These once handsome celebrities who have used surgical methods aren't quite as handsome as we once remember. Couple surgery and injections with laser and you might look a little freakish, not boyish.

Boyish good looks are a result of an athletic looking face - the words chiseled, toned and tightened describe an athletic looking boyish face.

Let's say you have decided not to use anything invasive or painful to maintain your looks and you realize that skin care doesn't keep your face, chin and neck lifted or tightened. Where do you go from here? You are the ideal candidate to learn facial exercise. Not contortions or girly movements but real isometric with resistance type movements that target specific facial muscle groups.

A work out for your face with simple yet effective muscle strengthening exercises can be completed in just about the same amount of time you need for a shower and shave. You don't have to go anywhere or wear special clothing; in fact, all you need are your thumbs, fingers and white cotton gloves in front of your bathroom mirror.

This specialized exercise routine targets fifteen areas of your face and neck and in hardly any time at all, from the inside out, your face will begin to resemble that boyish, younger looking you of years past.

Natural

Facial Exercise Is Green

"Green" became the world's best used buzz word with the advent of the new Millennium; this concept changed our consciousness forever. The shift in our thinking has affected the use of many everyday items we previously used without understanding the potential harm they wreak. Being more savvy consumers we no longer want shampoos, household cleaners, soaps, cosmetics and other daily used items filled with chemicals that affect not only our long-term good health but our every day living.

The move to use more natural ingredients has ingrained itself into our psyche as we insist that less chemical substances invade our bodies and living spaces. We opt for bamboo floors rather than carpet and paint that won't emit that strange smell. We are learning to adopt organic foods for the nourishment of our bodies and purchase products that enhance rather than compromise our lives.

The unrealistic expectations of plastic surgery procedures has produced a great amount of fodder in the tabloids not to mention a lot of disappointment for the men and women who have elected to use a very "un-green" method to in hopes of creating a youthful face and body.

Now as entertaining as watching celebrities slice and dice their faces, they, too, are rethinking their cosmetic surgery options. Gone are the days that surgeons acquiesce to the whims of their patients who want a Cindy Crawford nose, Angelina lips and augmented breasts that resemble a Baywatch Babe.

Injections that plump and paralyze became very popular a few years ago. The users of these injections didn't seem to mind initially that they were injecting their bodies with cadaver material, botulinum or chemicals that have no long term testing for efficacy. That is changing.

Maybe the state of the economy has swayed JQ Public's opinion but maybe those users are finding the futility of injections a big drain financially. Using expensive temporary fixes aren't a good investment and the results usually leave the users disappointed.

Facial plastic surgery could never be considered "green". In fact, plastic surgery cuts, pulls and sutures perfectly healthy skin just hoping that the user will find the results appealing and likable.

Plastic surgery is another futile attempt to sway the public that a barbaric measure can indeed help one look younger. Honestly, can you tell when a person has had a surgical procedure? Of course you can! Skin that has been altered never looks or acts the same.

Even facial peels that are so commonly used to lift dead skin cells are not considered "green". Why? Most peels, whether used in doctor's offices or purchased at your local drug or department stores are filled with chemical components and these chemicals can filtrate into the body's blood system.

Similarly injections that paralyze have long thought to migrate to the brain and other areas shortly after injecting; this migration may pose health threats. How green is that?

Green means honoring our bodies.

Exercise is one of the finest avenues to keep your body fit. Good nutrition enhances your body so eating plenty of organic vegetables and fruit will work to keep your body slim. Eating + exercise = better health.

Facial exercise is a component of exercise that has long been ignored. This very green method of exercise can produce results rivaling the finest face lift. Without sutures, without mistakes, without unrealistic expectations, your face can look healthier, revitalized and younger using simple isometric exercise techniques.

For years exercise has been thought to only affect the body from the neck down to the toes; however when your thumbs and fingers expertly hold and anchor the facial muscle or muscle groups, the result is a toned and tightened face.

If you are determined to live a more green existence, please consider using facial exercise over injections, electro-stimulation and surgery. You will love the results that are produced by exercising only a few minutes a day, people will easily recognize you and you will be so proud of your green accomplishment.

Is Your Face Man-Made Or Nature-Made?

Oh dear, it's true! Plastic surgery and injections that paralyze and plump are creating a world where those who have used these procedures have begun to resemble one another.

The "done" look is so prevalent especially in certain areas of the country where entertainment, music and fashion abound. The trickle down effect has begun to permeate the ranks of ordinary folk as school teachers, secretaries and wanna-bes go into debt to buy a piece of the American Dream that woos naïve men and women into believing that they too can look younger if they just allow certain procedures to be performed.

What nonsense!

Polluting the body, mind and soul with man-made chemicals and toxins that are then injected into various regions of the body means you are willing to forgo an authentic natural appearance and settle for the cookie cutter look that those injections produce.

The act of cutting and injecting produces the tell-tale look of face work and if you take a step back to consider the entire picture, these will seem like barbaric acts. After all, altering perfectly healthy tissue is pretty bizarre when you think about it. Most people who opt for procedures usually adopt an easy-breezy attitude as they conveniently forget that surgery and injections carry a lot of risk.

And, for those of you who use these modalities, do you really believe that your friends, family and colleagues cannot tell that your nose has been snipped, your eye lids cut and that injections have paralyzed your ability to genuinely smile?

Pretending not to notice an altered face may require great skill and tact. How do you gracefully react when you see a long-time friend who has obviously been sliced and diced? How do you stop from shouting, "What have you done to yourself!?!"

Many people undergoing procedures these days believe that job security will be enhanced when eyes are lifted and their double chin has smoothed. Those who have lost their jobs may be contemplating surgery and injections hoping that their new look will give them confidence in securing a new position.

Spending big dollars on temporary measures is not money well spent. In fact, surgery and injections do not provide long-lasting results nor are they guaranteed to provide the look you are seeking. These modalities constantly have to be upgraded because aging continues to permeate the face.

You can develop a younger, healthier, and fresher alive appearance as a result of incorporating a proactive regimen of exercise and paying attention to diet.

Exercise changes everything. We see our bodies respond when we bicycle, walk, row and perform other fun activities. Caring for your body temple is the first step in creating a more youthful you.

Exercise for our face is vitally important to our good health and spending only a few minutes each week performing certain isometric with resistance movements will ensure that you indeed look more fit, healthier and younger.

How does this happen? Those tiny, hidden muscles beneath the skin are the foundation of your facial appearance and when they become atrophied from disuse, they elongate and pool into other muscles as they make their way south.

You see the effects when hooded eyes, sagging cheeks and developing jowls make their presence known as you begin to resemble your great Aunt Hilda.

Using exercises that anchor and contract the facial muscles invigorates the various regions of the face with oxygenated blood. The skin, our largest organ, gets its nourishment from oxygenated blood while toxin removal and lymphatic drainage are two additional benefits your face will enjoy as it appears more relaxed, less stressed.

Facial exercise is easy to master and once you get your face in shape, you only have to exercise 2-3 times each week to maintain your results.

In hardly any time at all, your face will begin to transform by lifting and toning those areas you thought could only be remedied with surgery or injections. This natural facelift puts you in charge of your face without putting you in harm's way.

Men Want Real Women – What's a Woman To Do?

Did you know Katie Couric said "respect your wrinkles!" on NBC's Today Show? Matt Lauer said "confident women" are a turn-on and Al Roker agrees, "Women look sexy when they're just themselves, wearing jeans and a tee-shirt with less makeup."

They were discussing a poll released by Zogby International and ladies, men don't particularly care for the "Barbie doll look", rather from the 1,000 men who were surveyed, only 6% prefer Botox to wrinkles, 69% thought breast implants are not sexy and 50% want women to ditch the lipstick.

Then from Page Six, New York Post, April 26th edition, "You Sexy Thing!" based on a new poll by Zogby International says it's bad news for plastic surgeons because men prefer the natural look!

That's right - What men want and what they are looking for is changing! Most men aren't attracted to plastic, made-up women; instead, they want a natural, wholesome looking woman without the pulled, unnatural looking face most plastic surgery procedures produce, breast implants or Botox that paralyzes smiles and expressions.

Men want "real" women who aren't afraid to show off their God-given assets. They want women who will "say no" to docs who want to fill them up with Restylane, Botox and other dangerous substances that can harm and possibly maim the user long-term.

So, if men don't go for the Botox, breast enhanced implants, pulled face "Barbie Doll" look, who are these women trying to please? Themselves? Every time you choose surgery, you choose risk! Not just risk from the procedure but also the risk that men may think you less attractive!!!

What's a woman to do? How can a woman look and feel vibrantly younger without the "crutches" we've come to rely on?

Many people have been brainwashed to believe that when they experience facial aging, there's only one remedy - see the doc for surgery, laser, or injections. These temporary and very expensive procedures are risky; the patient believes they can buy a quick fix and then worry about the real aging later. Most patients do not realize that they're not prolonging the aging process with these procedures; rather they're masking aging in such a way that they will always be a slave to the next injection, a tweak here and there and most importantly, greater risk as the body compensates for foreign substances and healing requirements.

Trying to stave off Mother Nature is a very dangerous game when you try to fool her with unnatural means. After all, when one sees sagging, there are only a few options:

1) Do nothing and feel dowdy and old from your 40's onward

2) Spend your nest egg on injections, facial plastic surgery and lasers

3) Learn how to lift your face at home with a tried and proven method that keeps you looking younger and healthier day after day with no recuperative time, risk or financial burden.

Option #3 is by far the safest alternative because you can tone and tighten your facial muscles in only a few minutes a day. These muscles will contract, giving you a fresh, young appearance and your skin will look radiant from increased oxygen. You will have the look of a face lift without the hassle, the danger to your looks or general health or the expense.

You'll love your results – Promise!

Mess With Mother Nature and Sooner Or Later She Will Rebel

You have seen the look...shiny, taut foreheads, exaggerated lips, flat, moon-faced wrinkle-less or pulled, wind tunnel expressions that make you shake your head in wonder as you mutter to yourself, "What was she thinking?"

What she was thinking was that she only wanted a prettier face so that she didn't look old or feel ignored or invisible to a significant other.

Sometimes looking in the mirror at a face we barely recognize conjures up images of Great Aunt Hilda or Grandpa Joe or maybe we invoke disparaging names at our reflection as we commiserate our lost youth.

Beauty, many people believe, is purchased. Consumers go for most new lotions and potions offered in beautiful, slick magazines; they query one another at every outing to determine if they are up-to-date on the latest and greatest hype that separates them from their money. Walk by most any table with a group of gals and you will hear discussions of the steps they are taking to stave off the march of Mother Nature's footprints across their faces.

What is really alarming is the suggestion that beauty can be found at the end of a scalpel or the tip of a syringe bearing toxic paralyzing or plumping chemicals.

Sales of injections used as enhancements have skyrocketed in years past and new ones are being developed in laboratories worldwide right now. Even though discriminating individuals know these injections are laden with ingredients only a chemist could pronounce, they provide only temporary results that require refreshment on a regular basis. The cash outlay will add up quickly.

The side effects of toxic paralyzing injections used for frown lines in the forehead include nervous system disorders and drooping eyelids and eyebrows. What entices a user to use something that can make them appear older? It is a dicey decision.

In certain communities of the US the act of wearing a natural face without enhancements is almost an impossible feat. Why? The ads on tv, internet and magazines tout celebrities and because we long to emulate them, some of us do what they do. In a city such as Los Angeles where beauty rules, so do injections. Possessing a narrow vision towards true beauty, most practitioners steer their clients toward invasive procedures rather than natural methods because these modalities add dollars to their bottom line.

Keep in mind that 'facial improvements' are not always youth enhancing, some can be downright disappointing and these so-called improvements do not always look good on a 50 year old face.

Misshapen faces, overblown lips, eye lids that do not close and swept back cheeks are a result of Mother Nature's rebellious attitude towards unnatural methods that are risky and require recuperative time.

Quite possibly the more you fool with your face using products that do not support nature the greater the long-term damage. Consider a woman who visits an aesthetician, plastic surgeon or dermatologist; perhaps she only wants her face to look more radiant and she knows she is not ready for a face lift, just a little pick-me-up.

Most likely she will be enticed to participate in a series of facials first and then other anti-aging avenues such as micro-dermabrasion will be introduced.

Remember, the goal is for the client/patient to feel less than confident about their appearance, their age and aging so that injections, surgery, laser treatments and more can be offered.

If the client/patient opts for these expensive, temporary treatments, then the quest for the fountain of youth has begun at warp speed.

This heady trip of nips, tucks and high powered injections smacks Mother Nature full on and the delicate balance of our bodies begins to experience a life that relies on drugs.

Drugs have side effects and your body will likely rebel. The usual warnings such as redness at the injection site, slight tenderness or slight headache may only be the tip of the iceberg. What about infection, disfigurement and disappointment?

There is a way to look Mother Nature squarely in the eyes so that she supports your decision to look the best you can. There is a natural avenue that will maintain your face and it is called facial exercise.

Not contortions, twists, puckers or scrunches but simple isometric with resistance movements using only your thumbs and fingers in white cotton gloves that work to lift, tone and tighten sagging facial muscles that support your skin.

Plastic Surgery

Are You Too Old For Facial Plastic Surgery?

The jowls, the pouches, the hooded eyes looking back at you in the mirror are causing a huge drop in the confidence you once exuded. Here you are, middle aged to late adult and the aging you see in your face needs to be addressed if you want to look and feel on top of the game of life.

You know you will never look eighteen again nor will you have those rock hard abs and slim thighs that Matthew McConaughy loves in a woman but hey, you know you do not want to look like your Mom when she hit her middle stride or Great Aunt Helen when she developed the dreaded wattle that greatly aged her once beautiful face.

The smorgasbord of anti-aging choices may have you baffled. After consulting with those who specialize in plastic surgery, dermatology, skin care, those you love, friends who have had procedures and those who haven't; you now are armed with the latest and up-to-date arsenal of anti-aging procedures and methods that promote an illusionary promise to turn back the clock.

Yes, you want a younger looking face, but what's this? Have you waited too long to have a successful surgical facelift? Just how old is too old and these lists of complications and warnings, do they apply to everyone?

After the Donda West heart stopping tragedy, we now know that many men and women over the age of fifty have physical conditions such as issues with uncontrolled blood pressure, the beginning of heart disease, hematoma possibilities due to thin skin and previous health constraints that may create big red warning flags to a surgeon.

Previous surgeries, drug reactions, medications and even unrealistic expectations may prevent you from having a successful face lift surgery. Potential risks and complications that vary in severity are very real and you must proceed cautiously. Plastic surgery does not come with a money back guarantee and the results are permanent.

Even a simple eye lift may leave you dissatisfied with the results as you cope with swelling, eyelids that no longer close and excessive tearing. Infection and scarring are other risks that can present a challenge to your good looks.

Re-inventing yourself using surgery may not be for you.

Using injections also has drawbacks. Allowing foreign substances to be injected over and over year after year to plump and paralyze your sagging features may not always produce the desired effect as aging continues to affect the symmetry of your face.

Plumping up moderate not too deep lines and wrinkles is an art and when you choose injections you may not always like the results. Too, these temporary measures can have serious side effects that go far beyond redness and irritation at the injection site.

Perhaps surgery and injections are not appealing; the "done" look so prevalent in today's society might be right for some, but maybe not right for you. Benefits, precautions, adverse warnings and risks can be confusing.

An option that makes absolute sense if you really, truly desire a younger looking face is exercise. Facial exercise that uses resistance and contraction will slowly and steadily rebuild your facial muscles so they plump up. This action makes your skin look healthier; it acts and feels younger and smoother.

Just as exercise works for your body to sculpt and trim waist, tummy, hips and thighs, facial exercise can create a younger, more vibrant appearance when oxygenated blood is forced throughout the facial area. The face immediately begins to reflect the benefit of these exercises and every area of the face can be lifted, sculpted and refined with simple movements that are easy to understand and execute.

Will you look like you're twenty again? No, but if you want to look five, ten, even fifteen years younger, facial exercise is the safest procedure around. Think of it as a facelift without side effects.

Watch your face transform as the lines smooth and a youthful contour develops right before your eyes. You'll save thousands of dollars and never be at risk for the sake of beauty. Now when you look in the mirror, you'll want to say, "Well, hello gorgeous!"

Do Celebrities Regret Plastic Surgery?

What do celebrities such as Kathy Griffin, David Gest, Kenny Rogers, Jill Saward and others regret?

Do other celebrities such as Priscilla Presley, Cher, Joan Rivers and Melanie Griffith have the same regrets?

Are Michael Jackson, his sisters Janet and LaToya and Jackie Stallone related or do they, too, harbor regrets?

What do these celebrities have in common that causes them angst? Why, plastic surgery, of course!

Do you find it interesting that celebrities who can afford the very best surgeons and care often find themselves the butt of cruel jokes regarding their choices of using surgery and injections that were supposed to make them look younger?

Living in the limelight can certainly have its advantages and perks but there is a downside to living life on the red carpet and that is most likely why celebrities subject themselves to constant scrutiny that results in multiple procedures.

From nose jobs to breast implants, brow lifts to face lifts, cheek and chin implants, to eye lifts and regular use of Botox and fillers, the celebrity population keeps the plastic surgery business alive on both coasts.

John Q. Public loves celebrities and some even want to emulate them.

Just peruse any woman's magazine and you will find knock-off clothing suggestions from shoes, jewelry, sweaters, tops, slacks to coats coaxing the reader to look like a celebrity. Buying knock-off clothing and accessories to emulate a celebrity is just one step from wanting Jennifer Anniston's nose or Madonna's new cheek implants.

Aging with style and grace has been compromised with the advent of injections that plump and paralyze; add cutting perfectly healthy tissue, a very generous and sustained publicity blast that has kept these modalities forever in our psyche, and voila - faces are being cut, sutured, injected and altered at an alarming rate.

Do the procedures really help men and women to look younger and healthier? Do the risks outweigh the outcome?

Donda West and her untimely death easily comes to mind when you consider risks and benefits. Like Ms. West, many men and women in her age group have hidden health challenges that may not be uncovered until it is too late.

Choosing a well qualified surgeon is paramount; disclosing all medications, vitamin usage, previous health concerns and procedures will assist your health provider to determine your eligibility for plastic surgery. Choose a surgeon in good standing with the American Board of Plastic Surgery.

Plastic surgery is not a walk in the park.

Every surgery has its risks and dangers. Surviving a surgery then contracting MRSA (methicillin-resistant Staphylococcus aureus) is highly possible. This makes recovery especially difficult because eighty percent of facelift surgery infections are MRSA "Superbugs" according to a study conducted by researchers from the Lennox Hill-Manhattan Eye, Ear, and Throat Hospital and published in the Archives of Facial Plastic Surgery.

Other risks of cutting and suturing are that the results may not be what you anticipated. The skin surrounding the incision may not heal or act like your skin did previous to the procedure. Once healthy skin is cut, it is never the same. There is usually a loss of sensation (think Joan Rivers in the Geico commercial when she laments that she cannot feel her face) because the blood supply to the area has been diminished.

Injections that plump and paralyze do not always produce the desired results either. Too many visits with the syringe and you can begin to look freakish as taut and shiny are not synonymous with beauty and youth on a face that is trying to disguise old, wrinkled and droopy.

So what's the healthy solution for creating a younger looking face so the user doesn't have to suffer from invasive injections or risky surgeries?

The healthy solution is facial exercise. That's right, just as exercise works to trim, slim and tighten your waist, tummy, hips, thighs, torso and arms, facial exercises will address each slack, droopy facial feature and begin to systematically from the inside out tighten, tone and lift the areas that make you look old, tired and even lop-sided.

Facial exercises are more reliable than surgical procedures and injections because they can return your face to the look you enjoyed years ago. Your friends and family will easily recognize you as you present a fresh, pretty face for the world to see.

Exercise Stops the Need for Plastic Surgery and Injections

Almost every day there is an article written and published about the industry of beauty; the topics vary but you can be assured that Botox and fillers via injections, surgery and procedures will be discussed ad nauseam. These invasive, perilous undertakings entice those who want to look younger and these brave souls don't mind putting their health at risk as they alter their appearance time and again with the latest and greatest cosmetic procedure.

An unfortunate by-product of plastic cosmetic surgery is suicide. That's right, for whatever reason, men and women who are disappointed with the results are increasingly becoming suicidal. Body Dysmorphic Disorder (BDD) is real and its meaning can be summed up in just one sentence – This is a mental disorder suffered by both men and women that causes an extremely critical self analysis of one's physique with less than satisfactory results from plastic surgery or other modalities of physical enhancement. Imagine, having procedure after procedure and still seeing an ugly duckling in the mirror.

Chasing after the Fountain of Youth has been an on-going odyssey for centuries and even though drug companies would like you to believe that toxins and the like will help you look younger, at the end of the day, you will still be the age you are only with a body filled with chemicals that can have an adverse effect on your good health. This risk of dependency affects more than just physical health, now we must consider mental health!

Chemicals, toxins, cadaver based fillers, surgery, feather lifts, Thermage, lasers and more are temporary and risky procedures that keep you looking older. Yes, older! These fixes do nothing but prop up your aging face, producing short lived self confidence because when these gimmicks wear off, you must repeat and repeat the procedures to maintain the desired semblance of prettiness and youthfulness.

Does anyone who regularly shoots up think about the consequences ten years from now? It's a well known fact that when you paralyze a portion of the face, the face contorts to accommodate the affected muscles and these contortions lead to more wrinkles. What about the fillers that plump up nasal labial folds? How much can the body endure from repeated uses of sterilized cadaver and bovine materials?

And what about cutting into the face of a perfectly healthy body to stop the slide of muscles and skin? Consider this: If you see that your butt is sliding into the top of your thigh or that your underarm is jiggling, would surgery be your first line of defense? Heavens no! Most likely you would begin an exercise regimen to tone up your body; surgery probably wouldn't enter your mind.

Doctors and drug companies advertise. They heavily advertise so that you will begin to believe their message, their hype. They want you to believe that this injection, this procedure, this medication will make you look and feel younger and healthier. When you think about the long-term expense and risk, do these options seem sound? How many procedures and injections will be required over a twenty span? Will you eventually stop them and then just look old? That's doubtful because studies show that people who have one procedure will likely eye the menu and book another. It's likened to a gerbil on his wheel – imperfections can create the desire for more and more treatments that just might interfere with your life. After all, surgery is risky, even deadly!

I admire Alex Kuczynski, author of Beauty Junkies, who believes a very sad fate has tainted the feminine ideal, declaring that the culture of "better" has corrupted the perception of what is beautiful and even acceptable. In other words, the ads would have you believe that you need to be fixed. Ms Kuczynski nor I want you to end up look like an aging porn star from chasing after injections and surgery.

Enough already! Let's move on to a positive space – a space where everyone can return the look of youthfulness to their face without any risk, pain or spending their children's inheritance.

External beauty like inner beauty takes work; yes, it's easy to just allow someone to administer beauty enhancements but did you know there is an alternative to the usual suspects of improvement? One that will definitely help you look younger and it doesn't involve surgery or injections – it's facial exercise that uses isometric contractions and re-sistance that when employed for just a few weeks will create a younger looking face by strengthening and toning hidden facial muscles that support our skin.

Bottom line: Aging isn't what it used to be. Defy it! Exercise your face!

Facial Exercise Makes Plastic Surgery Obsolete

How old will you be when you notice the first signs of aging? Will aging affect your hips, thighs or buttocks first or will it attack your face, producing droopy eye lids and a sagging, jowly jaw line?

Think about this the next time you look at yourself in the mirror: When aging is apparent, what avenues will best serve you? Do painful injections around the eyes, lips and forehead entice you? Does it make sense to undergo a surgical procedure that promises you'll look ten years younger? Can you imagine waking up from surgery and not recognizing yourself?

Many men and women are searching for that special something that will keep them looking younger; taking vitamins, eating organic foods, practicing regular exercise, twice-monthly facials, are the norm for most health conscious people but no matter how diligent they are with a health routine, their faces continue to show decline.

Aging faces are primarily a result of sagging muscles; just like in the body where we discover our hips sliding down the back of our legs or the muscles in our upper arm looking loose and jiggle-ly, facial muscles suffer the very same loss of tone and resiliency. Add sun damage to the mix and all of a sudden you have an old, tired face that needs attention.

If indeed sixty is the new forty we're going to have to look long-term at avenues that are available to first stave off visible signs of aging and then correct the aging that has already become apparent. If you choose surgery, you choose risk. No matter how good the doctor, how qualified he is or where he practices; risks are present. Whether it's loss of sensation, slow healing time, infection or getting a look you don't necessarily care for, surgery, like injections is very temporary. Imagine spending $10,000 -$15,000 or more of disposable income and not liking the results or realizing that the aggravation and pain just wasn't accurately disclosed. Fast forward five years: most likely your face is in need of a tune-up and that procedure is going to set you back more money and again, put your health and well-being at risk.

Many people are beginning to understand that surgery should be the last resort when they've decided they've "had it" with a puffy, out of shape face, rather, they are opting for a safer and saner option. One that keeps them from spending loads of cash and doesn't risk their lives. That choice? Facial exercise!

You may find it difficult to believe that exercise can actually give the user a fresh, younger look but it does! Just as resistance and isometric exercise provides strength and toning for the limbs and torso, facial exercise will keep the face from sagging by tightening the muscles that support the skin. Your face will become more youthful looking as tell-tale aging melts away.

How is this possible? Muscles in the face are small compared to our other muscles in the body; the facial muscles attach at only one end to bone, the other end inserts into another muscle. Facial muscles weave over and under other muscles so when sagging begins, the muscles drop down into other muscles causing wrinkles and a misshapen face - the look of aging!

Stop aging now with easy isometric exercise. No pain, no surgery and no expensive, risky procedure to keep you a slave to unnatural methods.

How to Stave off Plastic Surgery Naturally and Attain a Younger Face

The world has seen great strides in medical miracles, technology and anti-aging. We see cutting edge conveniences everywhere as we live keep-up-to-date lives that have altered who we are.

We have cell phones that provide us with on-the-go communication as we download movies, music and news. Never in the history of our world have we been so closely connected as we further rely on the internet to bring us information, news, sports scores and more in real time – it's all readily available at our fingertips.

Preventing maladies and protecting our health has become everyday news. Anyone who reads, listens to radio and watches television knows that exercise and diet are vitally important to our good health; we choose our foods wisely and know that exercise improves not only our waistlines but also our blood pressure, blood serums and it keeps dis-ease at bay.

People seem to easily live healthfully into their 70's, 80's and 90's. Options for living longer means one can easily replace knees, hips, even elbows if they wear out; hearts and lungs and other organs are transplanted plus there are many, many drug and vitamin supplements that work to keep us vitally alive.

We live in a youth obsessed world. We don't want to feel old or look old; we want to look like the airbrushed models we see in magazines, billboards and television. Aging can be a painful experience as we look in the mirror and see an older face staring back at us. How and when did this happen?

Little by little facial muscles begin to lose their vitality. This loss of vitality produces noticeable sagging over time as the muscles elongate; this action drags the skin downward making one look tired, out of shape and old. One might see down turned mouth corners, a flabby neck or a lined forehead develop practically overnight. Aging in the face can alter our lives as we lose confidence in our appearance.

One option to turn back the clock is plastic surgery; it has certainly become mainstream and affordable but surgery has inherent risks such as anesthesia complications, loss of sensation, risk of infection and less than stellar results sometimes occur. Taking unnecessary financial risks and risking one's health to attain youthfulness is a very steep investment that one should carefully consider.

Another aspect of having a surgical face procedure is that muscles continue to atrophy, pulling the skin downward. Unfortunately, surgery does not stave off the aging process; procedures just mask the symptoms and the muscles continue to weaken due to inactivity. Surgical face lifts may be repeated and little "nips and tucks" performed periodically to "freshen" the lift; again, more risk for the patient.

Injections of "filler materials" have become so popular, one shouldn't be surprised to find them popping up in every airport kiosk. Botox® and Restylane® and Collagen are the "darlings" of the many available injections but they, too, only mask aging in the face. The results from these injections are temporary and must be repeated several times per year to counteract further muscle elongation.

What if one wants to proceed naturally? Is there a way to look revitalized when you don't want to spend money or risk your health to look younger and fresher?

There are those "weeds" and "seeds" - people who prefer everything organic and natural to achieve better health and they would never consider plastic surgery, rather you will find them seeking the latest information from their trusted naturopath and exploring other techniques that are proven and safe.

One easy way to a non-surgical, non-invasive face lift is to practice isometric facial exercise. This is a natural way to revitalize the facial muscles and yet look at least ten to fifteen years younger in just a few weeks. Isometric movements along with resistance techniques make a huge difference when you exercise your body; the same type of exercise will lift, tone and tighten the facial muscles. You will look healthier and younger as you laugh all the way to the bank.

Isn't Revision Surgery Just More Plastic Surgery?

A new industry within the industry of Plastic Surgery has arisen and it is called "Revision Surgery".

Under the Revision heading are many sub-headings but they have one thing in common: more surgery, more cutting of healthy tissue, more pulling, more tightening, more repositioning, more strings, more sculpting, more sutures, more injecting, more risks, more deaths and more dollars out of your wallet.

Revision Surgery is fixing things that went "bad" initially - bad nose jobs, bad breast implants, bad face lifts, bad brow lifts, bad eye lifts... you get the picture; think corrective surgery - fixing what hopefully can be fixed that got screwed up in the first place.

Some plastic surgery websites tell us that revision surgery is considered more difficult perhaps requiring a surgeon with a greater amount of skill and technique.

Plastic surgeons have never guaranteed their work so choosing to let another surgeon revise and correct the current unappealing physical situation may feel daunting.

It is.

Face lifts, brow lifts, neck lifts, eye lifts and more are very temporary fixes with permanent results. The altered face begins to sag after a few years and the patient must seek additional surgery, injections and laser treatments if they hope to look "normal".

Facial plastic surgery distorts the face over time and those muscles that once were sutured into place begin to lose their firmness and tightness; atrophied tissue is weak and this causes the facial features to unnaturally slide downward as they pool into other muscles and muscle groups.

This downward slide makes the face appear misshapen unless drastic revision methods are employed.

Facing more revision (elective) surgery will cost more than mere dollars. How are you guaranteed that you will like your results? What if you don't recognize yourself when you look in the mirror? What if your friends and family look at you in amazement thinking, "What has she done now?!?"

Opting for surgery is a big step that must be thoroughly weighed because once you allow cutting, you have forever lost your face in that you will never look like you again.

Oh sure, if surgery is needed to correct a malady, birth defect or physical challenge, it must be done. Using surgery to alter your appearance believing that this will make you look younger is flawed thinking.

Same with using injections that plump and paralyze. The reason you believe you need them is that the aging in your face is actually sagging facial muscles.

Loss of fat is the predominant cry but in actuality, the muscles that were positioned so perfectly when you were twenty five are becoming soft and mushy. This softening is creating the look of old.

If you have reached your fifties those once tight, well positioned facial muscles have now elongated about one-half inch so if you are wondering how those jowls and pouches arrived and set up camp on your jaw line, just know that the muscles around your mouth are slack.

It is the same with your eyelids. If your eye lids resemble crepe paper and they are droopy and saggy, this is a result of your forehead muscle elongating and pushing downward into the eye brows. This action affects your entire eye area as crow's feet become firmly etched at the corners of your eyes.

Blepharoplasty, eye lid surgery, has been very popular for over twenty years. As the forehead muscle continues to soften and elongate surgical revision after a few years is usually recommended because the eyelids continue to be affected with the gravitational lengthening of the frontalis muscle.

After a while you may begin to feel that you are like a gerbil on a wheel and that anti-aging is a very, very expensive process and extremely risky. Although initially one may look somewhat refreshed, there are always more procedures luring the susceptible and naïve patient searching for "the Fountain."

Long term use of procedures and injections may results in a freakish appearance that no amount of revision surgery can correct and if you want to avoid the gerbil wheel you may want to consider an all natural course of positive aging techniques to restore your facial features.

Using positive aging techniques such as isometric facial exercise puts you in the driver's seat and once you learn the movements, your face will look revitalized, tightened and lifted.

Each area of your face and neck can be exercised using your own personal "age erasers", your fingers and your thumbs. Learning to manipulate your facial muscles frees you forever from the need to use extraneous means to keep you looking younger.

Say no thanks to Revision Surgery and yes please to facial exercise!

No, It's Not eBay, But You Can Bid for Plastic Surgery

Desperate people can do desperate things when consumers become more savvy and sophisticated as they shop around for the very best deals offered on websites promoting surgical procedures.

That's right folks; you can offer a bid for that eye lift or tummy tuck on Bidforsurgery.com, just like you would bid on a piece of jewelry or camera equipment on eBay. If you select to pursue a bid, you are entitled to a free in-person consultation with the physician of your choice. This forum is designed to save the consumer time, money and effort thus saving the doctors administrative and marketing costs.

Insurance companies do not typically reimburse plastic surgery fees leaving the consumer to fend for the best deal with their hard earned cash. Prudent consumers can be thrifty and conservative when spending after tax dollars for a temporary face lift or other risky procedure that will undoubtedly need repeating in a few short years.

Another new wrinkle – no pun intended – was developed for the jet setting consumer who believes that they can enjoy a quiet surgical tweak in a foreign clinic where their dollar may go further because of low-cost, high-quality procedures. Sites like MedRetreat.com and PlanetHospital.com will book your appointment with a doctor then take care of the travel requirements such as passport and visas, airline tickets and hotel.

Life altering choices coupled with risk is a high price to pay for beauty especially when unrealistic claims and unqualified practitioners induce patients to make uneducated decisions. Even certain medical professionals are policing themselves and re-thinking their position on cutting into a healthy face for the sake of beauty.

Safety needs to be highly regarded for every surgical procedure and The British Association of Aesthetic Plastic Surgeons has published a checklist for those considering plastic surgery; it is the acronym entitled 'S.U.R.E.' We have seen similar admonitions from our US health officials and these are reminders of those warnings:

S: Surgeon's credentials and qualifications.

U: Understand fully the procedure, risk, location, downtime and care requirements.

R: Recovery process, how long, implications, after care options

E: Expectations can be over the top so be informed about what actually can be achieved.

All in all, warnings such as these are not needed when you use natural means to correct the cause of aging.

Some aging in the face is from outside influences such as over exposure to the sun and elements, smoking, drinking, poor eating habits, lack of water in the diet, too many adult beverages night after night, and the list can go on and on.

Some aging presents itself like sagging and this is caused when the muscles underneath your skin are elongating due to atrophy/disuse. The facial muscles, although small compared to say muscles in the forearm or leg, can cause noticeable aging when they begin to lose their shape and tone so by the time you reach 40, apparent aging has begun in your face.

Rather than opt for risky, temporary procedures such as injections and surgical treatments that tax your wallet, why not consider facial exercise to lift your face? You won't have to book an expensive trip or run the risk of contracting Montezuma's revenge or interview countless physicians hoping one of them can work with your budget and health constraints.

Exercises that use resistance and isometrics work for your body and the same principles can be applied to the face. It makes sense. Imagine seeing the face you had years ago returning day by day when you exercise your face.

The key to a younger, healthier looking face is prevention using a natural, safe method such as facial exercise to lift the sagging, droopy muscles without injections, harmful chemicals or cutting. Start now for a better looking face almost instantly!

The Funny But Not So Laughable After Effects of Plastic Surgery

Just when you thought it was safe to indulge your whimsical fantasies of a younger looking face using the latest and greatest plastic surgery techniques, you discover the tell-tale signs of injections and surgery to be blatant indicators of the ugly truth: these procedures can disfigure you and leave ugly reminders like scars, pits, unnatural lumps and bumps.

The injecting and over-injecting along with surgical missteps have caused a new vocabulary to evolve. Simon Crompton, a health journalist for 20 years, writer and editor, who has earned many acclaims, recently introduced the following maladies in his article The Real Perils of Plastic Surgery at Timesonline.uk:

BAT BROW

An injection of Botox in the correct forehead muscles makes them pull up drooping brows and eyelids. Hit the wrong muscle, though, and it pulls the brow down. Putting too much Botox in can give you a startled look, known as "bat brow", distinguished by permanently raised outer eyebrows, not unlike those displayed by Mr Spock. Fortunately, Botox wears off so the effect is usually temporary.

PING PONG FACE

There are around 140 injectable wrinkle fillers available in the UK and none of them are subject to the scrupulous testing required of medicines. Most are temporary, based on natural substances such as hyaluronic acid, that are reabsorbed by the body if something goes wrong. But there are also permanent fillers containing long-lasting synthetic substances, which can harden, cause obtrusive lumps and even move around. This week, 49-year-old Lea Martin spoke of how she had been left with an irremovable "lump the size of a ping pong ball in one cheek" after the injection of a permanent filler. Injecting too much filler can also result in over-inflation of the skin, known as "pillow face".

TROUT POUT

Because of the actress Leslie Ash, trout pout is probably the best-known cosmetic catastrophe; Donatella Versace and Pete Burns have also had it. Most cases of overenthusiastic lip plumping are temporary because natural substances such as collagen are injected. These slowly disappear from the lips into the body. The real and permanent problems occur when synthetic substances such as tiny plastic beads are injected, causing scar tissue to grow around them and becoming almost impossible to remove without scarring the face.

ROCK IN A SOCK

"Encapsulation" is the most common complication of breast enhancement surgery, occurring in about 10 per cent of cases. The body does not react well to an unnatural implant - it will try to reject it by becoming inflamed and then forming scar tissue around it, so the area around the implant becomes hardened. The problem can be especially bad in women who have had children and the breast is sagging. The implant pulls the breast down farther, and the hardened implant resembles a rock in a sock.

SKEWIFF EYELID

Hollywood celebs love an eye-lift, designed to tighten baggy lids above and below the eye. But surgeons admit that it is tricky. If the cut eyelid is repositioned incorrectly, it can turn slightly outwards and the eye becomes prone to running. Alternatively, the lid can become too tight if too much skin or fat is removed during the operation. Correction can involve inserting implants to stretch the skin.

TURKEY TUMMY

Removing too much fat with liposuction, or removing it too close to the surface of the skin, can leave the patient with dimples, irregularities, ripples and saggy skin. Many people who have lipo are not good candidates in the first place because they have too much abdominal skin - removing underlying fat only makes it sag more, leaving the midriff resembling a turkey's neck. "Smart lipo", which uses lasers to melt fat, reduces the problem by simultaneously tightening skin - to a limited extent.

POLLY BEAK NOSE

Badly performed nose jobs can result in unwanted lumps where the cut surface of bone or cartilage pushes against the skin. One of the most common deformities after rhinoplasty is called polly beak - as in parrot nose. It occurs when the surgeon, in repositioning the nasal cartilage, leaves too much at the tip of the nose, and a break occurs between the cartilage and the bridge of the nose - making it look hooked.

Mr. Crompton has nailed the pitfalls as he discloses that a group of disfigured cosmetic procedure victims have launched a campaign in the UK to better regulate the cosmetic treatment industry. These women hope others who have experienced botched procedures will step forward to join them.

Anti-aging serums, toxins and chemicals, eyelid surgery, breast augmentation and liposuction are a partial menu of services that have been financially rewarding for medical practitioners for many years. It is time for them to be held accountable so that we can remove Revision Surgery, a by-product of botched procedures, from our vocabulary.

Funny thing though...the procedures, whether injections or surgeries are risky at best. Just remember, things can go wrong very quickly.

Using Facial Exercise Means No Cutting or Injecting

In the quest for youthfulness John Q. Public has been the proverbial guinea pig.

It is true. For the past ten years or more injections that plump and paralyze have become the mainstay of many physicians including plastic surgeons, derms and now even OB/GYN's, dentists and proctologists have jumped on the cash cow bandwagon to fatten their wallets.

There is no end in sight even though warning bells have been rung to alert users that these injections may have hidden drawbacks with serious consequences that aren't readily identified.

Certainly the public has been warned that Botox migrates to the brain but what you may not realize is that if you choose certain plumping injections, you are receiving cadaver material that has been hopefully sterilized and then reconstituted so it can be injected.

Where do these cadavers come from? Are they the degenerates that fall dead on the street or drug addicts that donate their bodies to science?

Are you certain that the injections you are choosing will not have long-term ramifications that might prove injurious to your well being and good health?

Do you cringe when you read the list of possible side effects that you are asked to sign before receiving treatment?

Does it concern you that the injecting physician may not have adequately covered the list of contraindications or uncovered your medical conditions because you desperately want to stop nasal labial folds and your furrowed forehead?

Granted these injections can temporarily stop you from frowning and they can plump areas where folds and wrinkles have developed. Having these treatments once is not enough and in just a few short months, most likely you will begin thinking about repeating the injections as the plumping and paralyzing effects wane.

Let's say that you require two or three bouts of injections per year. Are you prepared to use injections for the next twenty or thirty years? Are you willing to spend thousands and thousands of dollars on temporary, dangerous fixes? Where does it end?

What if your health suffers and you are no longer a candidate for this type of intervention? Now what are you going to do?

Facial plastic surgery is yet another option that many people want to believe will keep them looking younger than their years, enrich their careers and lift their spirits. This is not necessarily so because many procedures will indeed alter your appearance but do you look younger or do you just look done?

Surgeries are permanent yet temporary.

You read that right. Even though your healthy face may be cut and sutured, the look of old will begin to creep back into the mirror as the real cause and culprit of an aging face has not been remedied or addressed.

Carefully study your face. What is it that makes you look old?

Do you see hooded eyes, concentration marks between your eye brows, jowls and pouches along your jaw line, a double chin or the dreaded wattle, cheeks sliding into your jaw so there is no distinction of contour, or nose to mouth lines and down turned mouth corners that resemble the marionette dolls of yore?

You probably see sagging muscles in your body in the form of loose skin in your upper arms, hips that are sliding down the back of your leg and an expanding waistline.

The real cause of aging begins with sagging, droopy, soft muscles.

When the face is affected by atrophied muscles the muscles begin to slide downward and pool into other muscles. This is when you see wrinkles and the look of old developing on your face.

If you are willing to spend a few minutes a day in front of a mirror, you can master a simple exercise routine that can produce the results you desire without resorting to costly injections or risky surgeries.

Most people want to look ten years younger and users agree that this is possible when using isometric with resistance movements. Slow, steady, consistent and deliberate actions can change the shape and contour of your face.

Without drugs or surgery or side effects you can indeed turn back the clock and look like you again with a toned, tightened and lifted face.

Could Those Nips and Tucks Speed Up Aging?

If you have tried facial plastic surgery, injections that plump and paralyze and liposuction for those hard to exercise places, you may be less thrilled with your results now than even six months ago.

There is news from a growing band of plastic surgeons, cosmetic doctors and dermatologists saying that cutting healthy tissue may indeed accelerate aging. This sentiment is not limited to just the US, this is an international concern being voiced almost daily.

Aging continues no matter what modality you choose. Let's say you opt for a surgical face lift; even though your facial muscles and skin have been cut and sutured, that tissue will continue its degeneration while adjacent tissue is also weakened from cutting and suturing.

This means you will notice sagging again and this sagging promotes tension in the surrounding tissue. Now you will be a candidate for the very popular "Revision" surgery that promises to fix the sagging, or does it?

Our faces "age" when the supporting facial muscles lose their shape and contour due to "disuse". This means that little if any movement you make with your mouth or face will keep those muscles taut and in good form. Over time the atrophy becomes noticeable as muscles and muscle groups pool into one another creating the look of lines, wrinkles and a sagging face.

Cutting perfectly healthy tissue as a "remedy" for facial aging means that the elasticity of the skin surrounding the incisions will be compromised and those muscles that were shortened and sutured will no longer have the needed volume that is present in a youthful face.

Cutting and suturing your beautiful face robs your skin of life-giving nutrients and oxygenated blood; instead of wearing the radiant soft look of youth, you realize that that you cannot fool Mother Nature. Cutting healthy tissue never improves the skin.

Facelifts have evolved with newer techniques; years ago, faces were simply cut, repositioned and sutured. Now the process requires that each area - skin, fat, muscle and fascia - be separated, individually repositioned and sewn while avoiding facial nerves that weave throughout the tissue.

Add muscle elongation to the mix of cuts and sutures, risks and dangers, and this is a recipe for the look of old and done and over done.

Disappointment and unrealistic expectations are genuine concerns of most physicians. Oh sure, they're trained on cadavers but surgery is not a definite art. There are human conditions and errors; sometimes there are health challenges and surprises that were not anticipated.

Dr. Michael Prager, a member of the Bristish Association of Cosmetic Doctors, is convinced from his clinical experience that anti-aging cosmetic surgery actually accelerates the aging process. He says, "Four out of five clients I see regret their decision to have anti-aging surgical procedures."

Surgery for any reason is risky and fraught with danger and should only be used as a last resort, especially on an aging face. Remember there are limitations to every surgery, the results are short-lived and the risks are considerable There are no guarantees that you will like the work or live to complain about the results.

Injections pose their own risk because injecting and injecting and injecting again may not produce the desired results long-term as the aging process will continue to affect the muscles in every portion of your face and neck. One pertinent question to ask is how many injections are you willing to have over the next 20 years and how much money are you willing to spend?

Another aspect of injections is the documented fact that these serums and potions can travel to the brain. That's right. When the face is injected with Botox, the risk goes beyond redness at the injection site; in fact, if you choose Botox, there is a long laundry list of health conditions and warnings you must sign off on to protect the injecting doctor and the drug company before anything is paralyzed.

Just remember that plastic surgeons aren't just pushing plastic surgery, now they have added injections and skin care treatments to their menu of services.

Fillers like Restylane, Collagen, Perlane and Sculptra have become popular to prop up sagging facial skin. Does everyone have a positive experience using these expensive, temporary fixes that dissolve into your system after a few months? Of course not. Are patients regretful? Sure, they are.

Alex Kuczynski, a reporter for the New York Times for eight years and now a columnist there wrote the fascinating book Beauty Junkies. In it she writes that she is not obsessed, okay maybe 'relatively' obsessed, but looking good at first meant 'maintaining'. Then she became addicted and tells how she had her first Botox shot at 28, spent over $8,000 in one year on microdermabrasion, collagen injections, more Botox and Restylane, an eye lift and other anti-aging modatlies. She decided when her top lip resembled a large yam after an unexpected Restylane reaction and much soul searching that that these methods did not ultimately add to her happiness and satisfaction and even labeled her liposuction foolhardy and wasteful. "No matter how much money you spend, or how much plastic surgery you have, or how many dermatologist visits you schedule, inevitably, times' winged chariot will catch up to you and march all over your face.'

We have read that Jamie Lee Curtis, Susan Sarandon, Julianne Moore, Jane Fonda and many more celebrities will not ever have more of anything plastic and instead have decided to age spectacularly. Here are these beautiful women plus others - who can easily afford the best of everything and they say no to procedures that could potentially wreck their health and their beautiful faces.

Will injections and surgery lose their status symbols as people realize that this type of self improvement is really self mutilation?

We want to look good for our age.

We want to feel confident and happy with our looks and we absolutely can without resorting to any life threatening, painful, expensive, temporary fixes.

The best choice to improve an aging face is facial exercise.

You want your face to look young and healthy, but how often do you exercise it? Just like body muscles that tighten with exercise, facial muscles that are stretched out, lax and droopy will respond to simple resistance training, too.

It is remarkable that by strengthening those tiny, hidden muscles with targeted exercise that this can act as Nature's facelift. You will feel the muscles respond immediately and this lifting, tightening and toning plumps up the muscles making the skin and face look younger.

It is wise to heed the docs who have seen first hand the effects of facial surgery, liposuction, facial injections, skin care regimens, lasers and products. Many believe that surgical cosmetic procedures can have a detrimental effect that shows up as thinning, discolored skin, hair loss and skin that just looks and acts older.

Facial exercise is the most positive step to recreate that younger face you thought you had lost forever.

Sagging Face

Can Facial Exercise Remedy Sagging Facial Skin?

Do you loathe looking into the mirror? Do you cringe when taking pictures knowing that photographs capture your aging face? Are you considering drastic measures or have you given up, thinking that your face will never, ever look youthful again?

A sagging, droopy face can make us feel old; never mind that all that talk about sixty being the new 40 if you are not happy with your appearance!

You may have discovered that no matter how many facial products you try, your face still looks old.

Oh sure, your face can look a little better after the latest round of dermabrasion and salicylic acid applications compliments of the aesthetician but you know that the problem you see requires more than just skincare.

More aggressive treatments seem necessary for sure.

Maybe you have considered using injections that paralyze - after all, your forehead is lined and mushy and your eyebrows are dropping. Your eyes look tired and eye makeup impossible to wear.

Yes, the recent horror stories nag at your confidence. Injecting a poison no matter how it is disguised via glamorous advertising does concern you and the recent disclosure of people dying from misuse of the serum along with the fact that no long-term test results have been forthcoming does makes you leery of this avenue.

Oh, but those nose to mouth lines! How can one possibly stop those without using injections that plump or cutting away the excess tissue?

Injections that plump are painful to endure and the results are so very temporary. Most likely you will spend a small fortune in the span of one year plumping and paralyzing your face only to have the very same to look forward to year after year. How many years can you safely use these products without long-term injury to the body? No one knows.

Counting on injections to keep you looking younger will leave you disappointed. Certainly you will see a difference in your face but after multiple injections year after year, your face may look misshapen. Here's why: No one really knows the long-term ramifications of injecting all these different potions into your face - how does the body dispose of these toxins and cadaver materials?

Doctors that inject are not magicians. They can get it wrong. The injections do not always produce the desired results of a younger looking face; rather, the opposite is possible. Instead of looking years younger, your face just looks injected and maybe unreal.

If injections are temporary, is surgery more permanent? Yes, the effect of surgery is definitely permanent but the aging process continues to escalate.

Just because muscles are snipped and sutured does not mean that your muscles stop drooping. Muscles support the skin and if they are in need of a tune-up, your face will sag even if you paid top dollar for a surgical facelift.

A face that has been altered by surgery does not typically age gracefully. The tell-tale unnatural slide of the muscles can produce small rows of cheek wrinkles - a look that indicates that the lift is sagging and in need of repeating if the wearer does not want to look old and bizarre.

Sagging facial features are a result of disuse. Disuse causes atrophy.

An athletic face on the other hand looks pretty remarkable and it defies aging. How? The athletic face is developed through specialized exercises designed to tighten, tone and lift sagging facial features.

Exercise changes the physiology of the body and exercise can shape and contour the face when contractions and resistance are employed using the thumbs and fingers in white cotton gloves that anchor the muscles. Without anchoring techniques, movements do not provide the necessary components that will impact the muscles positively.

From the inside out toned muscles develop and subtle changes work to make your face look and act younger.

Even if you have previously have had face work done, exercise will certainly maintain the lift and help you to stave off further surgery and injections.

Exercise changes the body and it can change your face so that you will look healthier and younger.

Facial Exercise Contours Sagging Facial Features

If you have looked in the mirror only to see the look of old peering back at you, you are not alone...your aging face began developing years before you celebrated your fortieth birthday. Those tiny facial muscles hidden under your skin contribute to aging when they no longer adequately support your skin.

At first you may not notice your facial features softening but slowly, very slowly the muscles begin to elongate and gradually your appearance shifts. Add sun damage spots, a few wrinkles around the eyes, wrinkles around your mouth, wrinkles in your forehead and all of a sudden you realize that Mother Nature has silently sabotaged your face making you look much older than you feel.

Oh sure, there are those who say that sun damage is the biggest culprit of aging and yes, it is wise to always protect your face, neck, back of neck, chest and the back of your hands daily with sun block - a preparation that has zinc oxide and titanium dioxide - but, muscles in the face elongate about one-half inch by the time you reach 55.

Elongation means one thing: your once uniquely beautiful tight face has developed soft, spongy muscles that no longer provide alluring contours. Rather, the drooping soft muscles are pooling into other muscles. This happens throughout our bodies as we see our derriere slide into our upper thigh and our arms develop bat wings. Blame inactivity and gravity.

Correcting sagging body muscles is usually accomplished via exercise; the very same principles of using exercise to reshape your body are applied to the face. Using strength building techniques that are easily mastered, an exercised face always looks years younger.

For years many people have opted for temporary modalities hoping that injections, lasers, thermage, surgery, electro-stimulation and deep peels would indeed rescue their sagging faces from further aging. Not the case...

The natural solution to facial aging is facial exercise. Unfortunately, these natural techniques have been skewed with misconceptions.

Ask the average Josephine on the street about facial exercise and most likely her reply will imply that facial exercise consists of scrunches, puckers and twists of the face. Ask Josie if she believes those types of movements will lift, tone, and tighten her face. It is likely that she is highly skeptical that contortions are a beneficial modality in her quest for a younger looking face. Smart gal.

Contortions, scrunches, puckers and twists will not produce the desired effects of lifting, toning, contouring and tightening droopy cheeks, dropping eyebrows and jowls, pouches or the dreaded wattle.

Creams and lotions will not shape, contour or tighten facial muscles. If you are wearing a turkey neck, (it is more than a sagging double chin), you are painfully aware that short of surgery and liposuction, there is no hope that your chin will ever look sleeker, more defined.

So it goes with the entire face and neck. What's needed is something that goes beyond topical skin care preparations, something that you can rely on, that you can trust and will work for you every time.

Resistance exercises use the body rather than weights to create a lean and toned look. Apply resistance training to the face and you will discover that your facial muscles become stronger but without bulk. They contour and reposition to give you back the face you thought you had lost forever.

To proficiently exercise facial muscles fingers and thumbs in white cotton gloves are used to gently anchor the muscles so that resistance is achieved while a contraction is created. Initially, this probably sounds a little strange but once you understand how this type of manipulation is accomplished, the movements will make perfect sense.

Your confidence will soar when the exercise movements are practiced six days in a row once a day for nine to twelve weeks because you will feel and see subtle changes each time you perform the movements. After six weeks of practice the results will last longer and longer.

So take a look in your mirror and assess your face. Does your forehead feel lax and mushy? Does your face look square? Do your mouth corners turn downward? Do you see jowls and pouches along your jaw? Have you ever lifted both sides of your face thinking you might need a surgical intervention? Does your neck look fat? Does it have loose skin?

If so, you will be delighted to learn that facial exercise will not disappoint. Facial exercises are the fastest, easiest, safest, least expensive and most powerful way to enhance your beautiful face.

Tighten Sagging Faces with Facial Exercise

Seeing a sagging, less youthful face looking back at you in the mirror can cause your psyche to do a double take ... all of a sudden your confidence leaves you as you realize that your jaw line is no longer firm and taut. You see slackness that cannot be disguised. The heavy, droopy eyelids, the cheeks that are sliding downward and that developing double chin are all tell-tale signs that age is showing on your face.

This scenario is very common. It happens to celebrities and it happens to ordinary people like you and me.

Many people succumb to the hype of surgery, laser and injections. They are more than willing to use artificial means to attempt to give Mother Nature the proverbial boot.

Usually when a person begins using injections to smooth, fill or paralyze fine lines and wrinkles, they have made a decision that will forever change their faces and perhaps even long-term good health. After all, do you really know all the ingredients in that syringe?

Having a needle stuck in your face every few weeks over and over, year after year, does not equate to aging well. Does it?

Preserving a youthful face has been the desire of most women and some men since the beginning of time. Creams, lotions, and other preparations have been used for centuries in hopes of curtailing the march of time across aging faces.

There are some pretty amazing topical skincare items in the market today but unfortunately they cannot stop the muscles from lengthening, dragging down and misshaping the skin and facial features.

Even after years of using the finest topical skincare products, skin loses its tone and elasticity resulting in an old looking, soft face. The muscles in the face attach directly to the skin so when the muscles become flabby from dis-use, the skin tone then is spongy and lifeless.

If you are like most consumers' surgery and injections scare you, and rightfully so; when aging is evident, sometimes desperate people take desperate means that fool with Mother Nature.

Wearing a healthy face – no sagging or droopiness in evidence is possible. Just as exercise is used to realize better muscle tone and sleekness in the body there are specialized resistance exercises that will produce the same type of results for the face.

Many good things happen to faces that are exercised. Increased circulation immediately de-stresses the features as the forehead, cheeks and eyes receive long needed lifting.

The most noticeable quality of an exercise face lift means tired muscles begin to plump up with oxygenated blood; the action of contraction affects the skin and it, too, feels and looks firmer and tighter.

The entire face and neck can be lifted, toned and tightened just like the body.

Take a look at your eyes. Hold a mirror at eye level and be honest: Do you see one or two tired, hooded eyes looking back at you? Do your eye lids feel heavy?

The very delicate area around your eyes can be traumatized by the weight of the forehead muscle pushing downward into the eye brows and then the eye lids. This compression causes crows' feet as the forehead muscle elongates into first the upper eyes and over time, the compression will affect the lower eyes as well.

Rather than fall prey to the hype that surgery and injections are the only options available, think exercise. Facial exercise will lift the sagging brows and forehead, create a wider area between the eye lashes and eye brows and put the sparkle back in your eyes.

Surgery and injections are not quick fixes. They are temporary at best. Recovery time and other issues such as infection, loss of sensation, disappointment, excessive bruising and scarring, nerve damage and prolonged healing need to be considered.

Exercise is natural, it's easy and the results will far out-rival the liquid or surgical facelift. Your face will look young and vibrant – your confidence will soar.

Seasonal

6 Don't Drop While You Shop Holiday Survival Techniques

1.) Get out of those tight fitting shoes

Shopping long hours requires comfortable shoes. When your feet hurt, the pain shows on your face making you look tired, irritable and maybe frumpy. Keep low-heeled comfortable shoes in your car and wear them when you're dashing around the mall looking for that hard-to-find compote Aunt Helen requested.

2.) Recharge your energy levels

The holidays are supposed to be fun-filled events that create long-lasting memories but if you're too tired to care, why not fortify your energy reserves with a potent vitamin combination of Vitamin C and potassium. Grab a glass of orange juice and a banana before you head out and feel positively super-charged for hours.

3.) Stop thinking sugar

Sugary foods will sap your facial beauty causing you to look with-drawn and gray. Cookies, cakes and candy are in plentiful supply every holiday season and if you give in to these temptations, not only will unwanted pounds linger on your hips, you may not look as sensational in that expensive dress you splurged on months ago.

4.) Grab your mate instead of your plate

Marathon parties equal too many calories and rather than chowing down at every event, grab your sweetie and get away from the food. Hit the dance floor, engage others in conversation, or try a sing-along; any activity that will keep your fingers out of the food will keep your figure in check come January 2nd.

5.) Not another glass of holiday cheer!

Overindulging in adult beverages can really pack on the pounds not to mention when you look in the mirror, your face spells d-i-s-a-s-t-e-r. A whirlwind round of parties can make your face puffy and older looking so a good rule of thumb this holiday season: For every glass of wine, drink two glasses of water to flush out those simple carbs.

6.) Keep up your exercise routine

Madly dashing around the mall may add steps to your pedometer but are you slacking off much needed cardio and resistance training that positively shapes your hips, tummy, waist and thighs? And, what about facial exercises that keep your double chin and hooded eyes from showing? By exercising from head to toe, you won't have to add "Start an exercise routine" to your New Year's Resolutions.

Summer's Coming – How Does Your Face Look?

Strappy sandals with colorful toe nails, tan limbs, easy-breezy haircuts, aromatic suntan lotions and wild-patterned beachwear. Ahhhh, summer!

There's a lot of preparation that goes into getting ready for summer.

Many people begin working out months in advance with a vengeance so they can sport toned, washboard abs, tighter thighs and hips and shapely arms. They carefully shop for the perfect outfits, shoes, bathing suits and revealing togs to compliment the newly sleek physique.

Getting ready for fun in the sun basically encompasses the region from the neck down to the toes and most people forget to include their faces in the regimen. Sure, they remember to slather on sun block, wear a hat and sunglasses, and are careful not to overexpose their bodies with too much sun but the fact remains that unattended faces can make one look older than their years.

An unattended face is droopy because skin care is not enough; there are jowls and pouches, thin unexpressive lips and usually a double chin or tired, lined eyes. Most people are unaware that exercise can work for the face just as it works for the body. Just like your body, your face has muscles under the skin and these facial muscles require exercise to keep the skin from dragging downward. When the skin loses its resiliency the facial muscles no longer support the cheeks, lower mouth or forehead and a misshapen face develops over time. Even lips will lose fullness as the face loses volume.

How does one recapture a youthful visage? Will creams, lotions and potions reverse sagging muscles and make the skin tighter? Only if they would; we could all have toned tightened skin on every area of our body. Just think about it...sagging underarms – no problem, let's just slap on a little cream or rear-end looking a little droopy – where's that magic potion? Alas, that's not possible.

Surgery for the face and lips has become epidemic yet there are many men and women who would rather count on natural methods to help them look their best. Nothing beats exercise. It forces oxygenated blood to the tissue, helps you look healthier and feel more alive. Imagine a younger looking face to match that new "ready for summer" body using an exercise routine that can be completed in just minutes a day. Not all exercise programs are created equal so for optimum results, choose one that offers isometric and resistance type movements.

In the face, the muscles are attached to bone on only one end; the other end inserts into another muscle or the skin. To achieve resistance the muscle and skin must be anchored. Only when the muscle is anchored can a contraction occur and when this happens, the muscle responds by tightening and repositioning; the face looks younger because the muscles, just below the skin, are in much better physical condition.

Skin

Facial Exercise Rejuvenates Tired Skin

Tired skin comes in many forms. It can be wrinkled, dehydrated, gray and lifeless. Without a doubt tired skin makes you look old.

Tired skin can be seen on various parts of the body. Sometimes your upper thigh may feel extra dry; it may resemble the Sahara Desert and treating the area so that it maintains its suppleness may seem challenging because wearing certain clothes next to your thighs can cause dryness.

Tired skin can sometimes be seen on the inner upper arms; perhaps weight loss has occurred, the arms could use weight training and just maybe, exfoliation is needed.

Tired skin can be seen on our faces and our necks, too. Sometimes our neck skin look dry, unattractive and very unhealthy; it can resemble dried out chicken skin.

Skin care advertisements permeate the web. They are everywhere! We see amazing photos that depict the most awful wrinkles, sags and bags that magically transform before our eyes as the 'before' face that was old and haggard now looks stunningly beautiful.

These fantastic results are not certified results but only Photoshopped images that capture our imagination. Nevertheless, these attention-getting hyped images provide a glimmer of hope and just maybe deep down we want to believe that there is a skin care item that could magically and easily erase the etchings of Mother Nature.

This type of advertised-sanctioned lying has become ordinary and it seems we come to expect it. Yes, science continually formulates concoctions to topically apply to our skin but there is just a lot of science fiction in advertising, especially on the web.

Tired skin cannot be enhanced with injections or even surgery. Lasers only resurface the skin temporarily as once again the wrinkles and tiredness will again begin to show as smiling, frowning and repetitive motions resume.

Chemical peels and micro-dermabrasion can remove old, dead skin cells; however, the lighter the solution, the lighter the touch, the less trauma to the skin.

Side effects are possible but by using a reputable, well-trained aesthetician will lessen the incident of long-lasting distress. Deep peels are more complicated and sometimes require anesthesia; there are risks with anesthesia and recovery time can take weeks.

Some of these methods can make your skin appear somewhat waxy, almost freaky looking and most people find this utterly unappealing. If you suffer from BDD, body dismorphic disorder, you may not notice that people talk behind your back, asking, "What was she thinking?"

Skin whether on our face or body is the largest organ of our body. Outwardly it is exposed to the elements and our skin reacts to what is going on inside the body. Skin can easily be attacked by bumps, hives, or other allergens. Choosing non-toxic topical preparations is important so that when the skin absorbs the lotions or potions, there is less damage internally.

Caring for the skin topically is important and learning how to care for it from the inside out requires a commitment for better health as you learn why choosing organic food, purified water and natural supplements may indeed provide a healthier lifestyle.

Dr. Nicholas Perricone, author of The Perricone Prescription, suggests we choose a diet rich in salmon, asparagus, lettuce, almonds, cantaloupe and lots of water to enhance our skin.

Facial exercise is the smartest choice for radiant looking facial skin. Our facial skin is supported by tiny muscles that weave over and under each other. They are attached to bone on one end and the other end attaches to either another muscle or it attaches directly into the skin.

These small muscles and the attached skin thrive and plump with increased oxygenated blood when the muscles are anchored in the right places using fingers and thumbs in exercise gloves. Simple isometric with resistance techniques slowly enhance the muscles in your face. The contractions that plump infuse the muscles and skin with newness.

These techniques contour the face so that the cheek muscles are more pronounced, the jowls and pouches lessen as they reposition up and back to the ear and the forehead strengthens lifting the brows recapturing your own beautiful facial features.

Facial exercise hardly takes any time at all. In the beginning you will spend only a few minutes per day learning and performing the movements. As you increase the routine and learn new exercises, in hardly any time at all, you will confidently breeze through the regimen.

The beauty of using exercise to look younger and produce more radiant skin is that there is no danger. Without chemicals, toxins or anything harmful, facial exercise will help your skin and face look youthful.

The Secret to Fresh Looking Skin

No matter the time of year, going out for the evening whether for dinner, drinks, dancing or just a movie, fresh looking skin is desirable.

Even if you have worked all day at home or the office, when it comes time to present yourself at night, you want to look fresh, vibrant and well rested.

Men have it easy - they can hop in the shower, shave, splash on a toner, finish with a moisturizer and voila - they are set for the evening. Women on the other hand require poofing and other subtle niceties that pamper their bodies and their faces.

Long, luxurious baths, loofas, and rich, hydrating potions cosset and coddle not only our bodies but our psyches as well. Going out for the evening is special and if we want glowing, radiant skin we must pay attention to our shoulders, arms, hands, décolletage as well as our faces.

The secret to better looking skin begins with daily routine maintenance that excludes harmful chemicals when we wash our hair and our bodies. Remember, your skin is the largest organ of your body and protecting it from excessive chemicals keeps you healthier longer.

Sesame oil is a wonderful substitute for chemically laden body moisturizers. Use organic oil from either your grocery or vitamin store (keep it only in glass) and apply it ten minutes before showering. It deeply penetrates the skin and what's most interesting about using this oil is that soap is not required. The yogis believe sesame oil possesses great healing power.

We definitely want to put our best face forward when we desire dazzling skin.

But what if your face looks gray, worn and tired? What if your eyelids are droopy and your eyes no longer sparkle? How can you perk up your cheeks without using tons of blush and ensure that your face glows with youthful radiance?

Making a last minute stop at the drug store to buy a new mascara or foundation hoping that these items will freshen your look will most likely leave you disappointed.

Brighter, younger looking facial skin is possible. Dullness is usually a result of an accumulation of old, dead skin cells - maybe decades worth so thick not even udder cream could keep your face moist.

Dermaplaning is an excellent way to remove dead cells that gray our skin; this procedure is performed by a professional such as an aesthetician or registered nurse. With a scalpel positioned at an angle to the skin, the back and forth motion certainly removes layers of dead, environmentally damaged skin cells. For most, this procedure is a luxury.

Daily at home care is vitally important if you want your facial skin to look healthy and bright. You can begin right now by adjusting your eating habits so that you consume a lot less sugar, more vegetables and fruit, hydrating your body daily with filtered water, using less alcohol and salt, regular exfoliation and exercising your face.

Facial exercise can lift sagging facial muscles. Exercise creates a radiance that is deeper than skin care and makeup. When you exercise your face, you will see and feel the difference immediately as oxygenated blood is forced through the tissues. You can actually feel the muscles respond to the lifting movements.

This all natural cosmetic enhancement has many benefits over surgery and injections; in fact, facial exercise is so reliable it makes plastic surgery seem barbaric.

Think about it - does cutting healthy tissue and then piecing it back together seem odd?

There is more than a healthy amount of trust required to allow someone to use sharp instruments to surgically alter your face. Your long term health could be adversely affected if there are unforeseen complications from excessive vomiting, over-use of prescription drugs, an undetected medical condition and more.

Even the finest surgeon cannot predict the outcome of your surgery or give you a money back guarantee if you are dissatisfied with the results. If you hate surprises, plastic surgery is not for you.

A word regarding serums that plump and paralyze; if you believe these expensive injections will stop your aging face, think again. Paralyzed and artificially filled faces continue to age. Do you really intend to fill your face and your body with unproven substances for the rest of your days? Your body may rebel resulting in sickness or even death.

Stick with facial exercise instead. You can easily develop the look of a natural facelift - one that does not require cutting, injections, sutures or recovery. The radiance you create will greatly become you as your confidence soars and your youthful face returns.

Fresh glowing skin isn't just for evenings now that you know the secret.

Why Skin Care is Not Enough

Staggering amounts of money are spent daily on cosmetics and skin care products that promise to lift, firm and tighten our faces. How many of us use a product for just a few weeks before purchasing yet another product? Do we jump from item to item because we really don't see a visible improvement and we feel disappointed in the results?

The ads are so compelling and we want to believe that we can look younger and healthier just by topically applying the latest and greatest discovery. Maybe that will happen one day but for most of us, using certain skincare items and cosmetic aids have not been helpful in the long-term because Mother Nature continues to tromp across our faces causing us to look older.

When we look at our faces in a mirror, if we're over 40, the aging we see isn't usually about wrinkles. The aging we see is looseness in our skin; maybe we see tired, sagging eyelids developing or a deepening nose to mouth fold or line. Our jaw probably isn't quite as distinguished as it was a few years back as it slides downward into the neck. Maybe this face is beginning to resemble your older relatives.

Is your face puffy and would you like to see it have more contours? No skin care or cosmetic product that can do that. Even dieting cannot produce the firm, toned, youthful face you remember in your 20's; in fact, dieting alone may deplete the fat underneath the skin making you look older than your years.

There are several avenues to address a droopy face but only one solution.

Many men and women seek plastic surgery to help correct signs of aging. Facelifts, eye lifts, and brow lifts are prevalent but they are only a temporary solution. The risk involved to one's health and bank account is dreadful. Infection, loss of sensation, slow healing time and unexpected outcomes are just a few potential complications one can experience from surgical procedures.

Another temporary avenue available is injected fillers that plump up the skin where there is creasing or a sunken appearance. Some injectables paralyze the muscles, relaxing the skin so wrinkles are less apparent. These expensive fillers are being injected at an alarming rate and the patients seeking treatments are younger than ever. Even though these fillers may temporarily ease the look of aging, the results will not last and will need to be repeated many, many times over a lifetime. These fillers only mask aging and the user will continue to experience sagging facial muscles.

So what is the secret to stop an aging face? It's exercise – Facial Exercise. Just like the body responds to Pilates, weight training, sit ups, etc., your face will look younger and healthier with exercise.

Just any old exercise won't do; isometric and resistance type exercises work for your face just like exercise works for the body. Facial muscles need exercise; the motions and movements we make daily aren't considered exercise because there is no resistance. No matter if you're singing, yawning or yelling; these movements aren't sufficient to create a younger looking face. The reason is that facial muscles attach to bone on one end and the other end of the muscle weaves over and under other muscles. It is only when special anchoring techniques are applied that a contraction can be caused in the muscle or muscle group; this contracting motion then allows the muscles to become fuller, plumper and more youthfully positioned. This action lifts the face.

Imagine applying these techniques for a few weeks and looking 10-15 years younger without invasive or costly procedures. You create the look of a face lift and save a ton of money with no risk to your health or your savings. You can keep the aging process in abeyance, feel revitalized, and look healthier and younger just by exercising your face a few minutes each day.

My name is Diann Kaufmann and I love what Facial Magic has done for me. One day I caught a glimpse of myself in the mirror and realized just how much I was beginning to resemble my mother. Don't get me wrong, I love my Mother, but at 48, I didn't want to look like her

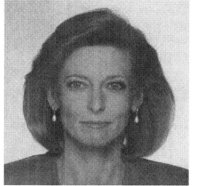

Then I began to seem invisible to the opposite sex, my confidence left me. About that time, a brochure arrived at my home describing a non-surgical method of correcting the areas of my face that concerned me; my cheeks were spongy, jowls were beginning to firm and worst of all, I knew people saw the bags under my eyes first. I kept that brochure around for days, reading and re-reading the text, and it all began to make sense to me. I had a feeling these specialized exercises for the face would work for me.

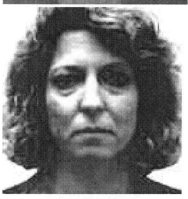

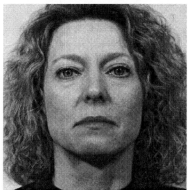

I began the Facial Magic program and in a matter of days, I saw subtle changes in my face. In weeks my upper cheeks began to develop in such a way that I had "high cheekbones". (The bones

had been there all the time but my sagging muscles prevented a more youthful look.) At the end of eleven weeks my entire face was firm, lifted and toned; most importantly, the bags under my eyes were gone! Facial Magic gave me a much younger appearance and I will use it for the rest of my life!

FACIAL MAGIC- "I am living proof that the exercises have helped me feel better about myself and that they do work."

You have a great product. I'm 43 and teach at SFSU - so I'm around very young & very old people. When I tell my students my age...(yes, the little buggers do ask)...they are often surprised. Patti, California

---

LUSCIOUS LIPS- "Give it a try."

Skeptical at first. I now know the Luscious Lips Pump has made my lips beautiful and definitely made fine lines around the mouth disappear. Give it a try! Helen, Ontario, Canada

---

LUSCIOUS LIPS - "Thank you for making a dream come true."

I am absolutely amazed at the results I had from using this device! It REALLY works! I am elated! I have wished for full lips since I was a little girl. I would not hesitate to recommend this to anyone. Thank you so much for making a dream come true. Rosalind, Birmingham

**LUSCIOUS LIPS - "...nothing makes lips as
sensual and youthful looking."**

We'd just like to say, as two really cool chicks, that for any woman (or man) who doesn't want to take the route of injection, NOTHING, and we mean NOTHING, makes lips as sensual and youthful looking (no matter what your age) as does the Lip Pump. Thank you! Babs & Reetz, Ontario, Canada

---

FACIAL MAGIC - "Facial Magic has enriched my life."

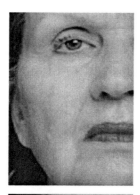
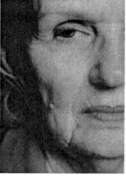

Facial Magic has enriched my life. The results I see in my face of firmness and texture truly give me a more youthful appearance. I love being part of the success of this product, for the integrity and truth for what it claims, but... most of all, I LOVE Cynthia Rowland. Her commitment to her program, together with her encouragement and dedication combine to make a youthful face possible for everyone. Yeah, Facial Magic! And, Yeah, Cynthia Rowland. Nancy O., Santa Monica, CA.

FACIAL MAGIC - "I love it and it certainly does work."

I've been using your Facial Magic system for about three years. I just love it and it certainly does work. Thank you. Joan W., Meaford, Ont. Canada

---

FACIAL MAGIC - "My hanging chin is gone."

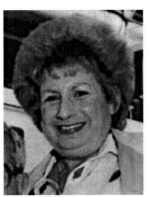
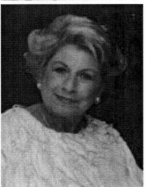

I am extremely pleased at what I see in the mirror when I look at my face. Lines along my forehead have disappeared. I can now see eye shadow between my eyelid and eye brow which I have not seen in years. It looks like I had an eyelift. My cheeks have plumped up near my eyes and heavy lines near my eyes are less. My hanging chin is gone. I can see a jaw line. When a neighbor of mine recently asked me if I had a facelift, I knew I was doing something right. Thanks for bringing Facial magic to me. It has given me more esteem than I have ever had. Bernice U. Tamarac, FL.

LUSCIOUS LIPS - "...I really don't think I could live without it now."

I really like the lip pump, and it gives my lips a much fuller and supple appearance. I use it in the morning before I put on my lipstick and it adds a lot more definition and fullness. My husband can really tell the difference. For anyone who has ever been self conscious of their lips or mouth it makes you feel confident. Thanks...I really don't think I could live without it now. Kelly

---

LUSCIOUS LIPS - "...my lips [look] fuller and younger."

Dear Cynthia, I wanted to let you know how much I love the Luscious Lips device. I am 54 and my lips look younger, fuller and more defined. I would recommend it to anyone. I have two daughters in their middle twenties and they both noticed that my lips looked fuller and younger. Thank you, Maria J. Hermitage, Tennessee.

LUSCIOUS LIPS - "I love the way my lips look after using the pump."

I have been using the lip pump for a couple months now and the results are great. I have had the collagen injections before but they don't last and they are very expensive.. The pump make the lines around my mouth plump out & hardly noticeable. I love the way my lips look after using the pump.. Thank you, Thank you.. Barbara L. Fremont, CA.

LUSCIOUS LIPS - "...the change in the size of my lips is incredible."

I've had the lip pump for about three months now, and the change in the size of my lips is incredible. I've always been self-conscious about having what I perceive to be thin lips, and have found the Lip Pump to be safe, quick, and with results that last for the whole workday. I feel a lot better about myself - a lot more attractive - and recommend this product to ANY woman who would like fuller lips but is wary of collagen injections and other more invasive procedures. Thank you very much for creating this product! Barbara V. Toronto, Ontario Canada.

LUSCIOUS LIPS - "UNBELIEVABLE"

As a makeup artist and former representative for a world-renowned cosmetic company, I feel confident in stating that there is nothing in the cosmetic marketplace that can enlarge the lips and help make fine lines around the mouth disappear (albeit temporarily) to the degree that the Lip Pump can. In brief: It has to be tried to be believed - UNBELIEVABLE, but is believable, because I tried it, and it works. Rita H., Toronto, Ontario, Canada.

LUSCIOUS LIPS - "...I can achieve really full, pouty lips when I want."

The lip pump device has been wonderful for me. I've never liked my thin lips and was tired of the expense and pain of collagen injections. My next step was going to be surgery before I heard about the lip pump. After several weeks of following the directions, I began to notice my lips looking much fuller. Now after using the device for several months I can achieve really full, pouty lips when I want. If you want full lips without the expense and pain of surgery please give the lip pump a try. I think you'll be glad you did. Monya.

LUSCIOUS LIPS - "I love Luscious Lips.."

I received the lip pump in the mail yesterday, and want to thank you very much for your help with my lip pump emergency! I have my device and feel human again (what does that say about me?). Anyway, thanks again. I love Luscious Lips and am telling all my girlfriends about it, and some of the guys too, though they just give me weird looks. Best regards, Barbara V. Toronto.

Product Ordering Information

Call Toll Free

800-592-3366

or visit our website at

http://www.cynthiarowland.com

You may also write to Cynthia Rowland

P.O. Box 3902
Long Beach, CA 90803

cynthia@cynthiarowland.com

9 780578 046693